The Health Disparities Myth

The Health Disparities Myth

Diagnosing the Treatment Gap

Jonathan Klick, PhD, JD
Sally Satel, MD

The AEI Press

Publisher for the American Enterprise Institute
WASHINGTON, D.C.

Distributed to the Trade by National Book Network, 15200 NBN Way, Blue Ridge Summit, PA 17214. To order call toll free 1-800-462-6420 or 1-717-794-3800. For all other inquiries please contact the AEI Press, 1150 Seventeenth Street, NW, Washington, DC 20036 or call 1-800-862-5801.

Library of Congress Cataloging-in-Publication Data
    Klick, Jonathan.
        The health disparities myth : diagnosing the treatment gap / Jonathan Klick, Sally Satel.
        p. cm.
        Includes bibliographical references.
        ISBN-10 0-8447-7192-9 (pbk: alk. paper)
        ISBN-13 978-0-8447-7192-2
        1. Health services accessibility—United States. 2. Medical care—Needs assessment—United States. 3. Medical policy—Social aspects—United States. I. Satel, Sally L. II. Title.
        [DNLM: 1. Delivery of Health Care—ethics. 2. Ethnic Groups. 3. Health Status. 4. Physician-Patient Relations. 5. Prejudice. 6. Race Relations. WA 300 K65h 2006]

    RA418.3.U6K65 2006
    362.1089—dc22
                                                          2005034903
10 09 08 07 06   2 3 4 5

Printed in the United States of America

Contents

Acknowledgments

The authors would like to thank the following individuals for reading all or parts of the manuscript and offering invaluable suggestions: Hal Arkes, Peter Bach, Doug Besharov, Ed Brann, Amitabh Chandra, Lisa Cooper, Barry Fogel, Michael Painter, Steven Schroeder, John Skinner, Philip Tetlock, Stephan Thernstrom, Amy Wax, and Lee Zwanziger. We are grateful to Sam Thernstrom, managing editor of the AEI Press, for his editorial excellence.

Introduction

I also come from Harlem, a community of poor black people. I've had the opportunity to study these people and . . . I find universality of discrepancies and differences. Race is not the issue. The issue is human conditions.

Harold P. Freeman, MD
Medical director, Ralph Lauren Center for Cancer
Care and Prevention, Harlem, New York[1]

Two fifty-year-old men arrive at an emergency room with acute chest pain. One is white and the other black. Will they receive the same quality of treatment and have the same chance of recovery? We hope so, but many experts today insist that their race will profoundly affect how the medical-care system deals with them, and that the black patient will get much inferior care. Is this really true? And if so, why? Are differences in treatment due to deliberate discrimination or other (less invidious) factors? This monograph critically assesses recent research bearing on these questions.

Interest in the determinants of minority health has grown considerably since the publication of the *Report of the Secretary's Task Force on Black and Minority Health* by the U.S. Department of Health, Education, and Welfare in 1985.[2] The academic literature falls into two categories. One line of inquiry emphasizes overt or subtle racial discrimination by physicians. Research reports in this category assert that many physicians treat their white patients

1

better than their minority patients on the basis of race alone. We call this the "biased-doctor model" of treatment disparities.[3]

The other line of research focuses on the influence of so-called "third factors" that are correlated with race. These factors can influence care at the level of the health system, the physician, or both. They include, for example, variations in insurance coverage (insured versus uninsured versus underinsured; public versus private health plans; profit versus not-for-profit health plans), quality of physicians, regional variations in medical practices, and patient characteristics (such as clinical features of disease, or health literacy).

Of course, it is possible that both of these mechanisms—biased doctors and third factors—could operate simultaneously. Practical policymaking requires an inquiry into the relative contributions of each. In our view, it is the third factors that generate the strongest momentum in driving the differences between races in both care and outcomes. Indeed, for answers to the race-related differences in health care, it turns out that the doctor's office is not the most rewarding place to look. White and black patients, on average, do not even visit the same population of physicians— making the idea of preferential treatment by individual doctors a far less compelling explanation for disparities in health. Doctors whom black patients tend to see may not be in a position to provide optimal care. Furthermore, because health care varies a great deal depending on where people live, and because blacks are overrepresented in regions of the United States served by poorer health care facilities, disparities are destined to be, at least in part, a function of residence.

Yet the biased-doctor model has acquired considerable and unmerited weight in both academic literature and the popular press. It enjoyed a great boost in visibility from a 2002 report from the Institute of Medicine (IOM), part of the National Academy of Sciences, called *Unequal Treatment: Confronting Racial and Ethnic Disparities in Health Care*.[4] The IOM provides lawmakers with advice on matters of biomedical science, medicine, and health, and issues high-profile reports written by panels of outside experts. *Unequal Treatment* was widely hailed as the authoritative study on health disparities. It concluded that the dynamics of the doctor-patient relationship—"bias," "prejudice," and "discrimination"—were a significant cause of the treatment differential and, by extension, of the poorer health of minorities.

Media fanfare greeted the IOM report in news stories bearing headlines like, "Color-Blind Care . . . Is Not What Minorities Are Getting" (*Newsday*); "Fed Report Cites 'Prejudice' in White, Minority Health Care Gap" (*Boston Herald*); and "Separate and Unequal" (*St. Louis Post-Dispatch*).[5] Virtually every story ran the triumphant remark of Dr. Lucille Perez, then president of the National Medical Association, which represents black physicians: "It validates what many of us have been saying for so long—that racism is a major culprit in the mix of health disparities and has had a devastating impact on African-Americans."[6]

There were a few dissenting voices. Among them was Richard Epstein, law professor at the University of Chicago. In his article "Disparities and Discrimination in Health Care Coverage: A Critique of the Institute of Medicine Study," he wrote:

> The IOM study adopts exactly the wrong approach. . . . Instead of dwelling [as the report does] on the Tuskegee experiments as evidence of current biases that linger within the system, I would trumpet the dedicated men and women in the profession who are determined to help people of all backgrounds and races deal with their health problems. . . . It is a shame to attack so many people of good will on evidence that admits a much more benign interpretation. . . . And there are enough problems in the health care system even without the genteel guilt trip that pervades the IOM study.[7]

But Professor Epstein was drowned out by numerous commentators who implied or stated outright that current treatment differences are a product of a harsh racial climate and personal bias on the part of physicians. To read David Barton Smith, for example, one would think it was only yesterday, rather than forty years ago, that we stopped segregating hospitals and separating the blood supply by race. There "remain key parts of the unfinished civil rights agenda," writes the public policy expert at Temple University, pending "enough federal will and national unity" to resolve them.[8]

In this monograph, we evaluate the studies routinely put forth as evidence of harmful discrimination. Because the IOM report represents the most popular synthesis of the disparities literature, we draw heavily on its analysis. We also examine evidence not considered by the IOM panel.[9] These additional findings indicate that race-related variables, especially geography and socioeconomic status, shine important explanatory light into the recesses of the treatment gap.

We conclude that the studies examined by the IOM panel—consisting primarily of retrospective analyses of large health-system databases—fail to make a persuasive case that physician bias is a significant cause of disparate care or health status. In short, the studies fall short in trying to control for the wide array of factors that confound the influence of race on physicians' treatment decisions. Without adequate controls, it is simply not possible to distinguish care patterns that correlate with race from those that are due directly to race.

Indeed, as we will see, when researchers employ designs that control for more third factors, the magnitude of any race effect shrinks considerably, if it does not disappear altogether.

Furthermore, we challenge the validity of measures commonly used to quantify health disparities and to calibrate the success of efforts to improve minority health. (We refer here to the assessment of *relative* care—that is, measuring the ratio of procedures or other health services received by minorities compared with whites.) One reason we question these measures is that the fact that a group receives more services does not necessarily mean it will have better health outcomes. For example, whites often receive more invasive cardiac procedures than blacks, but among blacks and whites admitted with heart disease, the death rate for whites is not necessarily lower.[10] Thus, if outcomes are the focus, blacks are not necessarily being undertreated. Instead, whites are perhaps being overtreated in some instances—given procedures that do not improve their prospects of surviving. Why might this be? It has been suggested that because whites are (or are perceived to be) more litigious, doctors practice defensive medicine with them.[11] In addition, whites are more likely to be insured, so doctors have more incentive to order additional tests.[12]

Second, the focus on relative differences masks absolute measures of improved care and thereby sends the wrong message to policymakers. For example, a 2004 study found that black patients with diabetes who attended a Bronx clinic were tested for diabetic control 53 percent of the time; whites were tested 57 percent of the time.[13] This difference of four percentage points could be considered smaller (and better) than the testing differential of fourteen percentage points found at a Washington, D.C., clinic. But a further look shows that 59 percent of blacks in the Washington clinic were tested, versus 73 percent of whites. In absolute terms, the D.C. diabetics—both black and white—received better care than their Bronx counterparts, but a narrow judgment based on racial comparison alone suggests otherwise.

Indeed, absolute improvements in treatment—if they occur in all groups—will not close a gap. All boats will have risen, so to speak. The minority group will have gained significantly, and good news this surely is; but the measure of success is obscured if one fixates on relative measures. For example, after the Department of Health and Human Services (HHS) implemented three-year (1999–2002) locally based projects in each state to help underserved populations overcome "healthcare system and sociocultural barriers" to care, evaluators found they could not document a reduction in statewide disparities, in part because the health of whites improved along with those of minority groups.[14] Although these projects were successful in improving overall community health, they failed to reduce racial disparities per se.

Conversely, a misplaced focus on narrowing of disparities can obscure deficiencies in care. Amal Trivedi and colleagues at Harvard, for example, found greater improvements in black patients than whites in receipt of required tests and treatments (for example, eye exams for diabetics or beta-blocker after heart attack) over a six-year period.[15] The good news about the narrowed black-white differentials, however, was somewhat offset by the fact that neither white nor black patients, all of whom were enrolled in Medicare managed-care plans, received the tests with optimal regularity.

Unfortunately, many scholars who address the disparity problem neglect the bigger picture. As David Mechanic, a world authority on health-care practices, laments, "Increasingly, much of the policy discussion is focused on whether disparities are increasing or decreasing and less so on which interventions can bring about the largest health gains for all."[16] He points to black/white infant mortality ratios as an example. From 1980 to 2000, black infant deaths decreased by over one-third, but because white deaths decreased more, the ratio of black/white mortality actually increased.

"Simply focusing on ratios misses important advances," Mechanic writes, "and may confuse us as to what is and is not worth undertaking."[17] In general, he points out, health conditions amenable to improvement through technology will inevitably benefit the most advantaged individuals and groups first because they have the knowledge, resources, and networks to gain access to them most quickly.

This is a powerful illustration of how a narrow concentration on race distracts from the reality that the largest overall gain in population health comes from targeting disparities linked to socioeconomic class.[18] True, race and class are intertwined and in some contexts can be proxies for one another, but they are both associated, independently, with health status. In fact, class makes a much greater contribution than race.

Consider the national data on mortality from heart disease. Adults in the bottom quarter of the income distribution are two to four times as likely to die from heart disease as those in the top quarter. The differences between blacks and whites are minor by comparison—the black death rate exceeds the white by only one-fifth.[19] And middle-class blacks are much less vulnerable to fatal heart disease than low-income whites. Put another way, controlling for income, blacks have higher mortality than whites; but low-income blacks have more in common with low-income whites than with middle-class or wealthier blacks. Thus, the socioeconomic differences between racial groups are largely responsible for disparities in health status between whites and blacks.[20]

The misplaced emphasis on relative care calls too much attention to the sensational but unsubstantiated idea that racial bias is a meaningful cause of health disparities. Not only is the charge of bias divisive, it siphons energy and resources from endeavors targeting system factors that are more relevant to improving minority health: expanding access to high-quality care and facilitating changes in individuals' lifestyles and their capacity to manage chronic disease. From this perspective, proposed race-based remedies for the treatment gap—such as racial preferences in admission to medical school, racial sensitivity training for doctors, and legal action using Title VI of the Civil Rights Act—become trivial or irrelevant at best, and potentially harmful at worst.[21]

Given the enormous political emphasis on racial disparities, we are compelled to respond to those who see treatment differences through a racial lens and design health-care policies accordingly. But a true public health solution to inadequate care—one that seeks to maximize the health of all Americans—would more properly target all underserved populations, irrespective of group membership. Success would be reflected in the improved health of these communities; and, because many of them happen to comprise large numbers of minorities, racial and ethnic care differentials would diminish as well.

1

Public Health Cast as Civil Rights

Just before Christmas 2003, the Agency for Healthcare Research and Quality, of the U.S. Department of Health and Human Services (HHS), released the *National Healthcare Disparities Report*.[1] It documented an all-too-familiar problem: the poorer health status of individuals on the lower rungs of the socioeconomic ladder, and the often inadequate treatment they receive compared to people with more resources and education.

The report sparked a heated controversy over whether HHS had downplayed the charge of racial bias in the health-care system. At issue were revisions made to a prepublication draft shortly before its release. Those included use of the more neutral word *difference* instead of *disparity* to describe discrepancies between the health of whites and minorities. This might seem like an innocuous substitution, but it was not. In public health circles, the word "disparity" has come to connote unfair difference due to a patient's race or ethnicity. It "has begun to take on the implication of injustice," observed epidemiologist Olivia Carter-Pokras at the University of Maryland.[2] Architects of the agency report, however, argued that the neutral term, *difference*, more accurately described their findings.[3]

The switching of *difference* and *disparity* prompted Henry Waxman, ranking minority member of the House Government Reform Committee, to send a harsh letter to Tommy Thompson, then HHS secretary. The word substitution, Waxman wrote, "alter[ed] the report's meaning . . . and fit a pattern of the manipulation of science by the Bush Administration."[4] The revision also set alarm bells ringing among a range of constituencies. "By tampering with the conclusions of its own scientists, HHS is placing politics before social justice," wrote members of the Congressional Black Caucus, Congressional Asian Pacific American Caucus, and Congressional Hispanic Caucus in a joint press release.[5] The National Medical Association pronounced itself "appalled."[6] Physicians for Human Rights bemoaned "remov[al] from the text [of] any inference of prejudice on the part of providers, and [its] focus on individual responsibility for disparities."[7]

The critics who scolded HHS for its revised executive summary cited the 2002 Institute of Medicine (IOM) report as proof that bias was common among physicians. While the IOM report did acknowledge the roles of other factors in minority health, it placed heavy emphasis on the failure of the medical profession to purge its ranks of prejudice—a shortcoming that was, as the report put it, "rooted in historic and contemporary inequities."[8]

Although the IOM report is now the most widely cited source for this claim, it was hardly the first to make the argument. A decade earlier, in *The Journal of the American Medical Association*, Secretary of Health and Human Services Louis Sullivan cast minority health as a civil rights issue, writing, "There is clear, demonstrable, undeniable evidence of discrimination and racism in our health care system."[9]

The Reverend Al Sharpton warned in 1998 that "health will be the new civil rights battlefront"; that same year, President Clinton remarked in a radio address delivered during Black History Month that "nowhere are the divisions of race and ethnicity more sharply drawn than in the health of our people," and speculated that one of the causes might be "discrimination in the delivery of health services."[10] In its 1999 annual report to Congress and the White House, the U.S. Commission on Civil Rights concluded that "racism continues to infect our health care system."[11] Recently, Senator Ted Kennedy urged that "greater resources should be given to the HHS Office for Civil Rights."[12] And, in an especially alarmist tone, Marian Wright Edelman of the Children's Defense Fund told the 2005 graduating class of Colgate

University that "the new racism that is seeping across our country is wrapped up . . . in racial disparities in health."[13]

We question the charge that episodes of doctor-patient miscommunication or assumptions physicians make about their patients are the product of doctors' ill will toward minority patients or disregard for them—sentiments implied by words like "bias" and "prejudice." Moreover, evidence (such as it is) that physicians' biased behavior is a major driver of disparate treatment is dwarfed by the undisputed and sizable effects of access to care and quality of care.[14]

Yet the social justice perspective often frames the issue of minority health. For example, introducing the Health Care Equality and Accountability Act in 2003, Senator Tom Daschle cited the need to correct doctors' "bias," "stereotyping," and "discrimination."[15] The American Medical Association felt moved to reaffirm its "long-standing policy of zero tolerance [toward] racially or culturally biased health care."[16] The American Public Health Association "call[ed] on the President and the Congress of the United States to recognize and promote legal redress for discrimination in health and health care."[17] On the research front, the National Institutes of Health are funding research on "the effect of racial and ethnic discrimination on health care delivery."[18] In some medical schools, "racial sensitivity" training is now required.[19] And, in 2005, New Jersey was the first state to pass a law requiring doctors to receive so-called "cultural competency" training as a condition of obtaining or renewing their licenses to practice medicine.[20]

These institutional mandates and practices legitimate the "biased-doctor model" of health disparities. We regret this, although we do believe that responsible clinicians should be aware of the potential for cultural misunderstandings between themselves and their patients. In fact, the IOM report may serve a useful consciousness-raising function, prompting doctors to ask themselves whether they are giving every patient the opportunity to benefit from treatment and to discuss complex issues, where appropriate, with them.[21] But, to the extent to which the IOM report is interpreted as evidence of widespread racial bias in the medical system, we believe its value is offset by the harmful consequences of this false conclusion.

Disparity: Difference versus Inequity?

The word "disparity" has various definitions, ranging in meaning from value-neutral imbalance to unfair and pernicious difference.[22] One of the earliest appearances of the term was in the 1985 *Report of the Secretary's Task Force on Black and Minority Health*, published by the U.S. Department of Health, Education, and Welfare (now HHS), where it referred to "excess deaths"— that is, the number of deaths observed in minority populations, subtracted from the number of deaths that would have been expected if the minority population had the same age- and sex-specific death rate as the non-minority population. In 1999, Harold Varmus, director of the National Institutes of Health (NIH), established a working group to address the problem of health disparities. That group was the first to devise an NIH definition of health disparities: "Differences in the incidence, prevalence, mortality, and burden of diseases and other adverse health conditions that exist among specific population groups in the United States."[23] Note that this definition is causally neutral, avoiding the question of what *produces* these differences.

The following year Congress established the National Center on Minority Health and Health Disparity. Its mission was to lead the NIH in its "effort to reduce and ultimately eliminate disparities," and assess its success in meeting the goal.[24] The center defined disparities as differences "in the overall rate of disease incidence, prevalence, morbidity, mortality or survival rate in a specific group compared to the general population."[25] Again, the language is silent on the question of causation.

Other government definitions reiterated the basic theme of neutral difference. For example, the *Healthy People 2010* report published in 2000 by HHS regarded disparities as "differences that occur by gender, race or ethnicity, education or income, disability, living in rural localities or sexual orientation."[26] And the Human Resources Services Administration, part of HHS, and the Minority Health and Health Disparity Research and Education Act of 2000, used the term to designate race-related differences in incidence of disease, access to care, or health outcome.[27]

Departing somewhat from cause-neutral definitions, the IOM report defined disparities as "racial or ethnic differences in the quality of health care that are not due to access-related factors or clinical needs, preferences and appropriateness of intervention."[28] While this did not necessarily mean that "bias," "prejudice," or "discrimination" must therefore account for differences in care that remained after "access-related factors or clinical needs, preferences and appropriateness of intervention" were accounted for, this was how the IOM interpreted them—an interpretation, as we will see, that was virtually preordained by the language Congress used to commission the report. In short, the IOM definition excluded every "good" reason for differences, so that only "bad" reasons were left. In his 2005 book, Thomas LaVeist, director of the Center for Health Disparities Solutions at Johns Hopkins School of Public Health, made the point sharply, defining disparities as "racial/ethnic differences in outcomes or quality of care that are indicative of injustice within the health care system or in the behavior of health care providers."[29]

Thus, with the definitional shift of "disparity" from being an observable difference to a moral failure, minority health was transformed from a public health issue into a civil rights issue.[30]

2

The IOM Report

As we've already discussed, the 2002 Institute of Medicine report was largely responsible for legitimizing the notion that racism among doctors is widespread. We do not believe that conclusion was well-founded.

In an interview on PBS's *NewsHour with Jim Lehrer*, Dr. Adewale Troutman, director of the Louisville Metro Health Department, illustrated the biased-doctor model well. Disparities, he said, have

> a lot to do with several factors, including what has recently been discovered as an issue of discrimination, potential racism, stereotyping and bias within the health care delivery system as defined by the Institute of Medicine report published in 2002. . . . And that may be a part of the answer as to why the black-white mortality gap has continued over these many years. But that particular aspect of healthcare that says that when you go into a provider, whether it's a hospital or an individual practitioner, and you happen to look a certain way—and there is a belief based upon the IOM report that there is provider attitude, whether it's conscious or unconscious and/or whether it's institutionalized racism that, in fact, dictates the kind of care that an individual is going to get.[1]

A strong claim—but is it true? We think not. There is insufficient empirical basis for Dr. Troutman's conclusion about physicians and his endorsement of the IOM conclusions. Before we address the nature and limits of the evidence put forth by the IOM, let us consider the ways in which its analysis and interpretation were influenced by its mandate.

The IOM report was commissioned by Congress in 1999 to determine whether differences in treatment exist when patients of any race or ethnicity have equal access to care. The panel was given two mandates. First, to "assess the extent of racial and ethnic differences in healthcare that are not otherwise attributable to known factors (e.g., ability to pay or insurance coverage)" and, second, to "evaluate potential sources of racial and ethnic disparities in healthcare, including the role of bias, discrimination, and stereotyping at the individual (provider and patient), institutional, and health systems levels."[2] The report panel, which comprised physicians, epidemiologists, social scientists, health economists, and administrators, commissioned additional outside experts to summarize peer-reviewed literature and government publications on health care and minorities.

In asking the IOM panelists to hold obvious determinants of treatment constant while having them focus on the potential "role of bias and discrimination" in health-care disparities, Congress practically invited them to interpret treatment discrepancies as evidence of bias. Simply put, if the IOM assumed that there were no benign explanations for disparities, then the only possible cause must be bias. Instructing the panel to hold major determinants of disparities constant had the effect of discounting them (and thus distorting the basis for policy recommendations). Because of these pressures, we believe, the panel erred in putting too much confidence in studies that were never designed by their authors to identify discrimination.

Missing Variables

The most rigorous studies reviewed by the IOM sought to control for confounding clinical or economic variables, such as concurrent illness, supplemental insurance, or patients' refusal to undergo procedures. But because most of the studies were retrospective and relied upon chart review or large Medicare administrative databases, many such variables could not be captured.[3] And as the

IOM report itself acknowledges, the more confounding variables were identified, the smaller the differential between whites and minorities became: "Almost all of the studies reviewed here find that as more potentially confounding variables are controlled, the magnitude of racial and ethnic differentials in care decreases."[4]

Some studies were more scrupulous than others in accounting for potential determinants of treatment, but even so, a treatment differential often remained. For instance, Saif Rathore and Harlan Krumholz (both of the Yale School of Medicine) identify four categories of information as potential explanations for differences in care: eligibility, contraindications, confounding, and patient preferences. Eligibility and contraindications refer to patients' clinical fitness for a procedure. Some of these variables are generally recorded, such as comorbid conditions and severity of disease at the time care is sought. Others are often missing from administrative databases—for instance, EKG subtleties, position of occlusion in carotid and coronary vessels, coronary ejection fraction, and pulmonary function test performance—even though they figure importantly in physician decision-making.

Moreover—and this is key—these unrecorded variables do vary by race and ethnicity. Note, for example, the well-documented frequency with which coronary angiograms of black patients show less anatomical suitability for intervention—either lesions in the vessels are too diffuse for angioplasty, or the patients have a higher incidence of normal-appearing vessels, despite the clinical appearance of having suffered acute myocardial infarction (heart attack).[5] An examination of records, therefore, could suggest a racial bias in treatment simply because coronary angiograms are less often given to black patients, and the records themselves do not indicate the reasons for those treatment decisions.

In addition to patient-level variables, other influential factors demand consideration. Geographical variations can occur, for instance, in practice patterns, quality of health centers, availability of subspecialists, adequacy of pharmacy stocks, or use of profit versus not-for-profit programs. There are differences in provider characteristics, such as qualifications or scope of providers' referral networks, and hospital-to-hospital variations in number of patients treated or procedures performed, on-site technology, nurse-to-patient ratio, and so on.[6] These dimensions went largely unexamined by the IOM panel because it relied on data from analyses using national samples that contained no geographic identifiers, or that based conclusions about the entire country upon data drawn from a single area or hospital. Further, other regional covariates, such as medical malpractice risk exposure, reimbursement rates, and managed-care enrollment rates, are necessarily excluded from these kinds of studies.[7] Even in studies that do control for regional variation, there are open questions about how finely regions have to be delineated to account for differences on the local level.

Consequently, the panel concluded that treatment differences occur everywhere, and that they are manifest for all kinds of care. But this conclusion was in error, as other studies indicate. Baicker and colleagues at Dartmouth College, for example, have shown important regional inconsistencies in treatment. One region might display wide race disparities in some procedures, such as hip replacement or back surgery, smaller discrepancies in bypass, and almost no gap in mammograms.[8] Does that mean that doctors in the region who perform hip replacements are biased, but cardiac-care doctors are not? Or is it possible that there are other, benign reasons for those statistical disparities?

Missing variables are not the entire story, however. Other kinds of evidence are necessary to bestow a fuller picture of the dynamics involved in treatment differences; without them it is difficult to have confidence in the IOM's claims about bias on the part of providers.

Prospective Studies

To perform an accurate assessment of the complex relationship between race and medical care, we need many more prospective studies that ask doctors and patients about how they make decisions to offer and to accept, respectively, particular treatments. The following vignette shows how difficult it is to interpret "bias" in medical records without an accompanying narrative from the clinician:

> Kathy A. is a nurse practitioner in a public health clinic near Washington, D.C. She treats many young African-American women. As part of the routine gynecological exam she asks them whether they had a PAP smear within the last two years. Typically, they say yes, and Kathy A. does not perform one. When she started looking through records systematically, Kathy A. realized that many of the women who said they had had a PAP smear never actually did. Soon she realized that many of the patients had mistaken a genital swab for STD for a PAP smear and has since kept this in mind during her history-taking (not to mention intensified her ongoing plea to the clinic director for computerized record-keeping).[9]

The innocent—though avoidable—mistake made by Kathy A. occurs daily in many inner-city clinics. On chart review, Kathy A. would appear to be a (white) clinician who was shortchanging black patients by not offering a routine PAP smear. But to allege that her error was borne of ill will, "prejudice," "bias," or "discrimination" is misguided. Indeed, asking doctors why they did not order a particular test could yield explanations such as the one offered by Dr. Gary Curhan. Writing in *JAMA* about workup for first-time kidney stones, he said, "If the patient is uninterested in making long-term lifestyle changes or taking medication, then I do not proceed with an evaluation [for a first stone.]"[10] Instead, he treats symptoms, like pain, but does not seek the cause of the stone. In other words, the physician decides to undertake an expensive workup only if a patient is invested in cooperating with the diet and other lifestyle changes needed to improve his condition.

Or consider the situation that confronts many nephrologists. As a patient progresses from stage four to stage five chronic kidney disease, the doctor or social worker is responsible for informing him or her of the options for renal replacement therapy. Ideally, the patient should be presented with three major options:

hemodialysis, peritoneal dialysis, or transplantation. Each of these has advantages and disadvantages, and patients are not equally suited for all. For example, patients with histories of poor compliance with treatment regimens might not be the best candidates for transplantation, since compliance with immunosuppressive therapy is critical to maintaining a functioning organ. In such a case, the physician or social worker may (consciously or unconsciously) present the options for transplantation in a way that "steers" the patient toward one or away from another.[11]

These examples highlight the social characteristics of patients as potential determinants of care. In his sweeping book, *The Status Syndrome: How Social Standing Affects Our Health and Longevity*, epidemiologist and physician Sir Michael Marmot documents the importance of factors that are not readily measured by disparity researchers—in part because their accounting requires time-consuming, face-to-face interviewing.[12] For example, Marmot emphasizes the importance of personal autonomy and control over one's life circumstances. With respect to treatment per se, it is not surprising that patients with chaotic lifestyles—an often inevitable aspect of living in or near poverty, irrespective of race— are not going to be good candidates for ongoing care requiring complex regimens.

Audit Studies

Without an experimental design in which all patients have equal access to the same range of services and expertise, it is very hard to know how to interpret differentials in care. An audit study, in theory at least, would help resolve this design barrier. Audit studies are highly controlled, labor-intensive investigations in which only one variable—race, in this case—is altered while access to a particular treatment, clinical appropriateness of the treatment, and patient desire for it are all held constant.

Unfortunately, there are very few audit studies of health-disparities research. Even more unfortunately, the findings of one of them have been badly misrepresented by its author. In 1999, Kevin Schulman and colleagues at Georgetown University School of Medicine published an audit study in the *New England Journal of Medicine*.[13] Briefly, the team made videos of black and white actors playing patients with chest pain. About seven hundred physicians viewed these tapes and were asked whether they would refer the patients to catheterization. The actor-patients were dressed in hospital gowns and described identical symptoms, had the same EKG findings, and the same health insurance.

Schulman himself erroneously stated to the press that the black patient-actors in the study were 40 percent less likely to be referred to catheterization, and explicitly attributed the discrepancy to bias.[14] The 40 percent estimate appears to have been based on a misapplication of statistics, as demonstrated by a recalculation of the Schulman data by a team at the White River Junction Veterans Affairs Medical Center in Vermont.[15] More accurately, white men, white women, and black men were referred at the same rate of 90 percent. The two black women actor-patients in the study were referred at a mean rate of only 80 percent, largely due to the low referral rate for one of them— probably a reflection of her unconvincing acting rather than anything else. In all, the probability of referral for all black actors in the Schulman study was 7 percent lower than for whites, not 40 percent. As the White River Junction team wrote in the *New England Journal of Medicine* several months after publication of the Schulman article, "These exaggerations [of 40 percent] serve only to fuel anger and undermine the trust between physicians and their patients."[16]

Though there ended up being little difference in referral rates, the Schulman study galvanized the press. Perhaps the most inflammatory report appeared on the ABC news program *Nightline*. Here is how Ted Koppel introduced the segment:

> Last night we told you how the town of Jasper, Texas, is coming to terms with being the place where a black man was dragged to his death behind a truck by an avowed

racist. Tonight we are going to focus on [doctors] . . . who would be shocked to learn that what they do routinely fits quite easily into the category of racist behavior.[17]

Race Comparison Between Doctors

A third kind of study valuable for understanding race-related factors in treatment compares care provided by white *and* black doctors to white *and* black patients. For example, evidence that doctors of both races treat black patients similarly, say, in terms of rate of referral for catheterization—even if both refer black patients less often than they do white patients—would cause us to question a charge of bias. We are aware of only one study that has analyzed data with this question in mind.

Jersey Chen and colleagues at Yale University analyzed data from the Cooperative Cardiovascular Project.[18] They evaluated forty thousand Medicare beneficiaries hospitalized for acute myocardial infarction in 1994 and 1995 to determine whether differences between black patients and white patients in the use of cardiac catheterization within sixty days after acute myocardial infarction varied according to the race of their attending physicians. Black patients had significantly lower rates of cardiac catheterization than white patients, regardless of whether their attending physician was white (38.4 percent rate of catheterization for black patients, versus 45.7 percent for whites) or black (38.2 percent versus 49.6 percent).

There was no significant interaction between the race of the patients and the race of the physicians in the use of cardiac catheterization, strongly suggesting that racial bias was not at issue. Critics of the Chen study, however, have suggested that the predominantly white cardiologists to whom the black internists referred their patients exhibited racial bias by undertreating the black patients.[19] To this Chen and colleagues reply by noting this would mean that black attending physicians concurred with and supported racially biased decisions—a scenario they believe unlikely.[20] Moreover, the adjusted mortality rate for black patients was lower than, or similar to, that of white patients for up to three years after the infarction, suggesting that the care received by the patients, even if it was different, was equally effective.

The mortality outcome in the Chen study raises an often-overlooked and somewhat counterintuitive point: Differences in care do not inevitably translate into differences in outcome. Granted, lower death rates (mortality) may not reflect less sickness while alive (morbidity). Indeed, Padma Kaul of the University of Edmonton and colleagues did report evidence of poorer functioning within six months of acute myocardial infarction for black patients due to their lower rates of bypass surgery compared to whites.[21] Nonetheless, it is not always safe to assume that not undergoing a procedure inevitably causes harm. We should not reflexively interpret these differences as signs of inferior treatment.

The results of the RAND Health Insurance Experiment—a landmark study conducted between 1974 and 1982 to discover how much more medical care people will use if it is provided free of charge—are instructive. By randomly assigning subjects to different insurance arrangements, the researchers were able to prompt different levels of care and expenditures unrelated to the subjects' underlying health characteristics. By and large, the RAND research suggests that, in many contexts, increased treatment and expenditure levels do not translate into systematically better health.[22]

Outcome Studies

Chen's finding of comparable mortality for blacks and whites is by no means unique. In fact, according to a Kaiser Family Foundation review of cardiac care studies, the overwhelming majority found no mortality differences between races despite lower rates of procedures for blacks.[23] Writing in *Medical Care* in 2005, Amber E. Barnato of the University of Pittsburgh and colleagues found that black patients had a lower risk of dying within thirty days of admission to treat acute myocardial infraction than clinically equivalent white patients at the same hospital. They observed this pattern despite the lesser likelihood of black patients receiving invasive care.[24] A 2005 study in the *New England Journal of Medicine* examined almost six hundred thousand "ideal candidates" for cardiac procedures from the National Registry of Myocardial Infarction from 1994 to 2002. Though white men underwent reperfusion (for example, balloon angioplasty or clot-dissolving treatment) more often than other groups, the thirty-day in-hospital mortality was no less for them than for black men and white women.[25]

One possible explanation is that catheterization may be overused in white men, meaning that the procedure is performed even when it will probably not benefit patients, because, as suggested earlier, doctors are practicing defensively to avoid liability.[26] Thus, higher frequency of invasive medical intervention and rates of coverage do not inevitably translate into better health.[27]

Recently, however, the pattern has been changing, showing greater mortality for blacks after acute myocardial infarction. Skinner and colleagues found a greater ninety-day mortality in a nationwide Medicare sample, which they attributed to the fact that the care of black patients was concentrated in hospitals that provide lower-quality care.[28] As Marc Sabatine of Harvard Medical School and colleagues demonstrated, though, quality of inpatient care is not the sole explanation. In his study, blacks and whites received similar protocol-driven care, yet six-month mortality was higher among black patients.[29] The authors speculate about the roles of "multiple socioeconomic and cultural factors undoubtedly at play."[30]

Discerning the rate of use that represents the highest quality of care is essential, because the remedy for differing rates of treatment due to unnecessary care in one group will not be the same as that for discrepancies based on underuse of needed care in another. The overtreatment of whites, however, can still coexist with the undertreatment of minorities. Researchers at Albert Einstein College of Medicine examined this possibility explicitly by analyzing New York State Department of Health data for 12,555 patients admitted to New York City hospitals with heart attack. They found that whites had higher rates of angioplasty and bypass grafting than blacks (25.2 percent versus 15.8 percent), though death rates during hospitalization for both groups were comparable. The death rate among blacks who did not receive bypass was similar to that of whites, suggesting that blacks were not inappropriately denied access to the procedures. Data on complications and course of recovery were not reported.[31]

When access to care is good and quality of care and patient characteristics are relatively uniform—such as in military health-care systems—racial disparities in care after controlling for the extent and severity of the disease are negligible.[32] A number of studies have documented comparable use of cardiovascular, pulmonary, and oncological procedures in black and white patients treated by the Veterans Affairs medical system.[33]

Others have shown similar or slightly better mortality rates for blacks compared to whites, despite receipt of fewer interventional procedures, such as catheterization and endarterectomy.[34] Notably, neonatal and infant mortality was found to be equal for white and black babies born to parents enlisted in the military; in the general population, black infant deaths are at least twice as frequent.[35] Suggested explanations for these phenomena include greater access to care and follow-up visits; more similarity between races within the Veterans Affairs patient population compared to the general population in terms of income and medical comorbidity, health-related attitudes, and higher quality of care; and monitoring of standards at Veterans Affairs medical centers affiliated with medical school and residency training programs.[36]

Thus, there are many explanations for the treatment gap. More of the kinds of studies just described—detailed prospective studies, audits, black-white doctor comparisons, and outcome analyses— are necessary to better understand physician decision-making. Nonetheless, many medical schools, health philanthropies, policy-makers, and politicians are proceeding as if physician "bias" were an established fact. In the following chapters we explore additional possible explanations for health disparities for which studies need to account.

3

Bias?

The claim that physicians' "bias" or "prejudice" toward minority patients is a fundamental dynamic driving health-care disparities is explosive—but we believe it is unproven and improbable and, as we have discussed, distracts from other factors influencing the nature of care patients receive. In the end, inferences about bias basically come down to an absence of sufficiently clear benign explanations for differences in care. Theoretically, this makes sense, but in practice no studies that we are aware of meet the burden of accounting for the panoply of factors that influence care. From a research standpoint, then, bias is largely a diagnosis of exclusion.

Thus, when studies find a persistent treatment gap after attempts to account for some of the obvious variables, we are left in ambiguous territory with much room for speculation. This is why it is imperative that researchers who are trying to identify bias within the doctor-patient interaction define their terms clearly and weigh alternative hypotheses.

According to popular understanding, bias may be conscious or unconscious in origin. Conscious bias underlies a knowing act—a deliberate effort to disadvantage members of one group solely because of who they are.[1] Unconscious bias, on the other hand, denotes an automatic or "implicit" assumption based on race or ethnicity. If the assumption is unflattering—for instance, that the patient will not adhere adequately to treatment, is not well-educated, or abuses alcohol—it is called negative stereotyping.

Saif Rathore and Harlan Krumholz have noted vagueness in the use of the term "bias." They cite a "lack of framework" for interpreting reports of variations in health-care use by race and ethnicity but finally conclude that "racial bias with adverse consequences in health care may be inferred if a racial variation in treatment . . . persists after accounting for health care system factors."[2]

Economists Ana Balsa, Thomas McGuire, and Lisa Meredith have attempted to parse the mechanisms by which treatment differences can result from an encounter between a doctor and patient.[3] The authors identify three mechanisms. The first and most blatant is overt prejudice. The prejudiced doctor would, presumably, be unwilling to treat patients from the disfavored group, either by avoiding practice in certain communities altogether or deliberately spending less time with them during visits. If he were required to treat them, he might give inferior care. The other two mechanisms, labeled "uncertainty" and "stereotyping," are kinds of inferences that arise from the mental shortcuts doctors routinely take in the face of incomplete information.

Balsa, McGuire, and Meredith recognize two versions of uncertainty. The first is miscommunication. This arises when the doctor has difficulty interpreting a patient's report of his symptoms: Individuals in same-race doctor-patient pairings, it is suggested, understand one another better than those in mixed-race ones. In turn, poor communication leads to differential care, with adverse outcomes for minorities. The authors call this "statistical discrimination," based on a concept first elaborated in the workplace, wherein white employers have an easier time assessing the productivity of white workers. (This is somewhat different than the standard definition of statistical discrimination, which means making a determination about an individual based on the average attributes of his group.)

The other form of uncertainty is called "rational profiling." This is a decision-making shortcut normally used in the presence of ambiguous or inadequate information. Here, the doctor knows from his own experience or the medical literature that the frequency of particular health problems and the effects of treatments can differ across races. Thus, he will consider medically relevant probabilities associated with race in diagnostic and treatment decisions—an example being the faster progression to renal complications in blacks with high blood pressure than in hypertensive whites.

Stereotyping, according to Balsa, McGuire, and Meredith, is another decision-making shortcut. It involves the reliance of doctors on negative assumptions about individuals from minority groups. Much-cited examples are found in studies by Michelle van Ryn and colleagues, wherein physicians were presented with clinical vignettes and asked to make inferences about patients of different races portrayed.[4] Despite similarity of information provided, the authors found that doctors were significantly more likely to expect black patients to dismiss medical advice, to be less likely to comply with rehabilitation, and to be more likely to abuse drugs and alcohol.

The distinction between rational profiling and negative stereotyping does not strike us as sufficiently clear—after all, some unflattering assumptions may simultaneously be rational ones. Balsa and colleagues seem to be blurring the distinction between factual judgments and value judgments or moral assumptions. Generalizations about compliance, for example, especially by a physician who is well-acquainted with the clientele of his community, may well be factual *and* negative. Though poor compliance is an undesirable characteristic in a patient, that doesn't mean the doctor inevitably dislikes his noncompliant patients or will treat them less competently.

Consider Dr. Neil Calman, an internist at Albert Einstein College of Medicine in New York City. In an essay in *Health Affairs* subtitled "A White Doctor Wrestles with Racial Prejudice," Dr. Calman flagellates himself for his "prejudice," which surfaced when he began caring for a black patient named Mr. North.[5] Dr. Calman describes being made to feel "vulnerable" during the first visit by Mr. North, who, the doctor knew, had been recently released from jail. The patient towered over him, spoke in a deep bass voice, and did not remove his reflecting sunglasses. It turned out, contrary to Dr. Calman's expectations, that Mr. North was highly conscientious about his health, kept all his appointments, and maintained careful records of his myriad medications. This surprised Dr. Calman, and he felt guilty about that. But that does not mean his assumptions about the patient were entirely unfounded, or that he was prejudiced. He felt uneasy during the initial visit because Mr. North was, in fact, acting like an intimidating ex-convict. And despite his unease, there is no evidence that the care he provided Mr. North was diminished by these feelings. Dr. Calman had worked for a quarter-century as an inner-city family doctor who, in addition to giving high-quality treatment, regularly took on social work tasks—for instance, finding a home for the children of one his patients, a single mother dying of AIDS. If this compassionate, devoted, and introspective doctor is "prejudiced," as he calls himself, we clearly need more like him.

Thus, we question whether negative assumptions about patients are the automatic equivalents of prejudiced attitudes (classically defined as hostility and rigidity and erroneousness). After all, unfavorable impressions can simply reflect realistic group differences in patterns of disease and behavior and imply nothing about the moral disposition of the person who holds such an impression. Indeed, if the doctor's assumptions are unaccompanied by ill will, are paired with efforts to compensate for an unfavorable perception of the patient (such as of poor compliance), and are amenable to change as the doctor sees, for example, a particular patient becoming more conscientious, then is this really prejudice? What harm has been done?

For example, if a physician assumes that a patient will not comply with triple therapy for HIV and simply forgoes the medication, he has acted unethically—even if he feels no ill will toward the patient. But giving the patient a compliance "trial," wherein the patient must at least keep a second appointment in order to receive medication, or assigning him to a special nurse-manager who phones him with medication reminders—even if it turns out that the doctor was wrong in his prediction of poor adherence—does not strike us as biased.

Furthermore, we are skeptical that doctors, or most decision-makers for that matter, act on inferences based on race alone. At the very least, key elements in the doctor's reasoning surely include observable phenomena as well: the patient's general demeanor and degree of engagement with the clinical exam and history-taking, for example, complemented by the doctor's experience with him. A patient who sees the same doctor from visit to visit has the benefit of preservation of clinical information and the opportunity to establish a rapport with him.

Negative stereotypes, in the end, may best be addressed through the self-correction that comes from calling attention to their existence. Journal clubs (weekly gatherings of medical professors and trainees to discuss newly published research) and bedside teaching rounds are good venues in which to develop the habit of being mindful of the complexity and subtlety of clinical discretion and assumptions made within the doctor-patient relationship. Compared to classroom settings, which have their place, rounds-based discussions offer a more organic way of addressing the issue because it is incorporated into day-to-day clinical routine.

To our knowledge, there exist no systematic, prospective evaluations of physician decision-making in relation to patient race, let alone of the clinical results of such decision-making. The literature on medical stereotyping contains data that are indirect, limited to interpretation of academic exercises that may have heuristic value but are inadequate for drawing conclusions about actual clinical encounters.

4

Is Geography Destiny?

If bias is not a driving force behind differences in health care, what is? With most health care delivered locally—and with racial and ethnic groups not evenly scattered about the country—it is imperative that researchers account for geography in evaluations of health disparities. When they do, they discover that geographic residence often explains race-related differences in treatment better than even income or education. One of the most striking limitations of the IOM report is the absence of such an analysis.

Consider the concept of the "hospital referral region," or HRR. *The Dartmouth Atlas of Health Care* defines an HRR as a geographic area served by a major hospital equipped with comprehensive surgical capacity, also known as a tertiary care hospital.[1] In the United States there are 306 HRRs, yet only 36 of them have a nationally representative mix of residents. Among the rest, a number have black population rates that are three to six times the national average of 13 percent (see figure 1). Because health care varies a great deal depending on where people live, and because blacks are overrepresented in regions of the United States that are burdened with poorer health facilities, disparities are destined to be, at least in part, a function of residence.

Medicare datasets do not include geographic identifiers, so geographic data are often lost to researchers who rely on these sources. Consequently, as Amitabh Chandra and John Skinner of Dartmouth College have observed, many disparity evaluations do not sufficiently control for geographic variation among patients.[2] This can produce misleading findings.

FIGURE 1

Distribution of Black Residents Nationwide

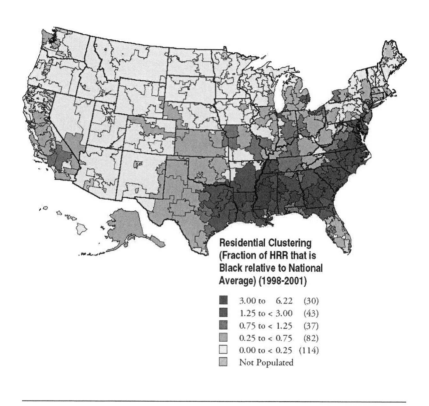

Residential Clustering
(Fraction of HRR that is
Black relative to National
Average) (1998-2001)

- 3.00 to   6.22   (30)
- 1.25 to < 3.00   (43)
- 0.75 to < 1.25   (37)
- 0.25 to < 0.75   (82)
- 0.00 to < 0.25   (114)
- Not Populated

SOURCE: Chandra and Skinner, "Geography and Racial Health Disparities."

For example, assume black patients from two different cities—city X and city Y—receive exactly the same care as white patients from the same places. In city X, all patients receive suboptimal care; in city Y, all patients receive excellent care.

Now compare the care of all black residents of cities X and Y with the care of whites from both cities. If the proportion of black residents in the two cities is not identical, there will appear to be racial differences in treatment even though blacks and whites living in the same place receive the same care. Thus, if minority patients are not randomly distributed throughout locations—only 6 percent of poor whites live in high-poverty neighborhoods while 22 percent of Hispanics and 34 percent of blacks do— geographic differences in utilization and health outcomes are going to appear, analytically, as racial disparities.[3] And researchers who fail to control for location effects will interpret geographic health disparities as racial disparities.[4]

As a rule, the quality of care received by blacks is inversely related to the concentration of black residents in the local population. For example, Baicker, Chandra, and Skinner found that the frequency of annual eye exams in black diabetic patients covered by Medicare declined as the number of blacks in the local population increased.[5] Along these lines, blacks who lived in predominantly white HRRs received the same or slightly better eye care than whites. Angus Deaton of Princeton University and Darren Lubotsky of University of Illinois have found that at both the regional and the metropolitan statistical area (MSA) level, both white and black mortality rates are higher in areas where blacks make up a larger portion of the total population.[6] Similarly, the Dartmouth group found significantly higher risk-adjusted mortality following acute myocardial infarction in U.S. hospitals that disproportionately serve black patients.[7] In her study, Amber Barnato and colleagues found that 1,000 of 4,690 hospitals nationwide accounted for treating 85 percent of the black Medicare patients in 1994–95.[8]

The effects of location on health disparities have also been studied using infant mortality rates. Jeannette Rogowski and colleagues at RAND used the rich Vermont-Oxford network dataset to examine the effects of hospital quality on the mortality rates of very low-birthweight babies, controlling for condition of the baby at birth (via Apgar scores) as well as other characteristics such as gestational age, race, method of delivery, birth defects, and prenatal care.[9] The authors found that black babies were more likely to be born in hospitals that primarily served minority areas (57 percent for black births, as compared with 18 percent for white births).

Thus, at a minimum, black and white babies are not being delivered at the same kinds of hospitals. The characteristics of the hospitals serving these two populations also varied systematically. Black babies were significantly more likely to be born in government-run hospitals that served a relatively high proportion of Medicaid patients, and where doctors spent less time with patients due to high patient volume (and for other reasons as well). Further, the hospitals where black babies were born were significantly less likely to have neonatal intensive care units or to perform neonatal cardiac surgery.

In the Rogowski analysis of twenty-eight-day infant mortality rates, these hospital characteristics proved to be a significant source of variation in the survival chances between white and black babies. Babies born in minority-serving hospitals were 30 percent more likely to die in the first twenty-eight days than those born in hospitals that served few minorities (less than 15 percent of patients), and this effect was quantitatively similar for both white and black babies.

Although not nearly as important as the minority-serving versus majority-serving distinction, many other hospital characteristics that differed by race also proved significant in determining mortality. For instance, having a neonatal intensive care unit that performed cardiac surgery reduced infant mortality by 14 percent, and being born in a government-run hospital raised mortality rates by 7 percent relative to a private, not-for-profit hospital, and by 24 percent relative to a for-profit hospital. Again, these results included controls for condition at birth, prenatal care, maternal income and education levels, and gestational age.

Thus, by focusing on race we miss a very important cause of health-care difference: geography. Where a person lives has a much larger effect on how the medical system treats him.

5

Role of Hospital Variation

As we have seen, regional differences in health care can be a significant factor influencing health disparities. Variation among hospitals is another factor for which disparity studies often do not control. Indeed, the studies below describe a pervasive trend: Hospitals that treat greater numbers of minority patients generally offer poorer quality service than those that treat fewer minorities.

In general, hospitals that perform a low volume of surgical procedures such as coronary bypass, gall bladder removal, or valve replacement have higher mortality rates for the given procedure than those that perform more. A 2002 study by John Birkmeyer and others showed that black patients were more likely to be treated at low-volume hospitals and more likely to die for that reason.[1] The crucial importance of volume has been underscored by the Leapfrog Group (a coalition of more than eighty large public and private insurance purchasers), which urges both patients and payers to select hospitals that perform a certain minimum threshold number of procedures per year.

Elizabeth Bradley of Yale and colleagues found that hospital-to-hospital differences made a considerable impact on treatment differentials in the case of suspected heart attack. The cohorts included 37,143 patients receiving angioplasty at 434 hospitals, and 73,032 patients receiving fibrinolytic therapy (medicine to dissolve blood clots in coronary arteries) in 1,052 hospitals. Their findings: "A substantial portion of the racial and ethnic disparity in time to treatment is accounted for by the hospital to which a patient is admitted, in contrast to differential treatment by race and ethnicity inside the hospital."[2]

Within the region of New York City, Lucian Leape of the Harvard School of Public Health and colleagues found that about one-fifth of all patients who needed balloon angioplasty or bypass graft did not get them, largely because the hospitals to which they were admitted did not have onsite catheterization labs.[3] The frequency of failure to recommend these procedures and to transfer patients to sites at which they could be performed was equal across racial groups. Moreover, when patients were admitted to hospitals with onsite facilities, there was no racial variation in the rate at which the procedures were received.

Another study of New York State examined surgical complications by race. Using the 1998–2000 New York State Inpatient Data Set, a team led by Kevin Fiscella of the University of Rochester found that black patients had higher overall rates of postoperative complications, especially thromboembolism (blood clot) and septicemia (infection). When they controlled for patient-level characteristics (for example, presence of additional medical conditions) and hospital features (size, number of full-time registered nurses), racial differences in complications were "fully explained."[4]

Blustein and colleagues at Columbia University assessed the frequency with which whites and blacks patronized poorly equipped hospitals.[5] Following a cohort of 5,857 patients admitted to California hospitals with acute myocardial infarction in 1991, the authors found that white patients were more likely than blacks to travel past community facilities that lacked catheterization laboratories to tertiary hospitals that had the technology available.

A nationwide study of all Medicare patients treated in 4,690 hospitals between 1994 and 1995 for acute myocardial infarction (heart attack) revealed a similar finding. On average, black patients went to hospitals that used evidence-based medical treatments (that is, state of the art practices) less frequently and had worse mortality rates (but higher rates of cardiac procedures, suggesting better-quality surgical than medical care). "Incorporating the hospital effect altered the finding of racial disparity analyses and explained more of the disparities than race," wrote Amber Barnato of the University of Pittsburgh and her coauthors.[6]

Once again, we find that minority patients receive different treatments than whites primarily because they attend lower-quality hospitals—a pattern that helps exonerate physicians from the charge of systematic bias in their treatment of patients. Most likely, this is a function of minorities' disproportionate poverty or near-poverty status. Studies comparing similarly disadvantaged blacks and groups of whites (such as those clustered in poverty in Appalachia and rural Maine) would underscore the primacy of social capital (such as education and wealth) over race in the receipt of care.

6

Impact of Malpractice

Financial risk associated with doctor malpractice insurance—and its impact on physician workforce distribution throughout the country—is another factor in access to care for minorities. Jonathan Klick of Florida State University and Thomas Stratmann of George Mason University examined the effects of medical malpractice reforms on where doctors choose to practice over the period 1980–98.[1] They discovered that states passing caps on noncompensatory damages in medical malpractice cases were more successful in attracting doctors. Additionally, the increase in the number of doctors practicing in these states appeared to have the largest effect on underserved communities with large minority populations.

This shows that when medical malpractice litigation risk grows, the doctors who consider moving to another state in response to that risk tend not to be those serving affluent, predominantly white communities. Doctors most sensitive to this risk (and the concomitant increase in liability insurance costs, as well as financial risk in general) are those with more modest incomes who are serving or considering serving marginalized communities.[2] Consequently, liability protections should improve access to care for individuals in these communities.

Klick and Stratmann go on to show that damage caps passed by the state translate directly into improvements in the black infant mortality rate. This is because doctors now have more financial incentive to practice in underserved areas. The authors found that enacting caps on noncompensatory damages at the $500,000 level reduces the black infant mortality rate by sixty-seven deaths per hundred thousand births, a statistically significant result that implies a reduction in average black infant mortality of about 7 percent. Increased access is likely to help both white and minority residents alike, but because the minority residents make up a disproportionate share of the population in these underserved areas, the effect will be to provide relatively greater improvements in minority health.

These results are consistent with other research examining the effects of increasing access to prenatal care generally. Lisa Dubay of the Urban Institute and colleagues found that decreasing doctors' exposure to medical malpractice liability risk increases the likelihood that mothers will receive prenatal care early in their pregnancies.[3] Though this effect is statistically significant for both black and white mothers, the magnitude of the effect is much larger for black mothers. Daniel Kessler of Stanford University and colleagues also reported that tort reform increased physician supply.[4]

7

Patterns of Physician Use by Race

A central assumption that underlies the biased-doctor model is that black patients are served less competently than white patients by the same (white) physicians. But research by Peter Bach and colleagues at Manhattan's Memorial Sloan-Kettering Cancer Center and the Center for the Study of Health Care Change in Washington has produced findings that cast doubt on that assumption.[1] The authors showed that white and black patients, on average, do not even visit the same population of physicians—making the idea of preferential treatment by individual doctors a far less compelling explanation for disparities in health. They show, too, that a higher proportion of the doctors that black patients tend to see may not be in a position to provide optimal care.

The research team examined more than 150,000 visits by black and white Medicare recipients to 4,355 primary-care physicians nationwide in 2001. It found that the vast majority of visits by black patients—80 percent—were made to a small group of physicians—22 percent of all those in the study. Is it possible, the researchers asked, that doctors who disproportionately treat black patients are different from other doctors? Do their clinical qualifications and their resources differ?

The answer is yes. Physicians of any race in the study who disproportionately treated black patients were less likely to have passed a demanding certification exam in their specialty than the physicians treating white patients. More important, they were more likely to answer "not always" when asked whether they had access to high-quality colleague-specialists, such as cardiologists or gastroenterologists, to whom they could refer their patients, or to nonemergency hospital services, diagnostic imaging, and ancillary services, such as home health aid.

These patterns reflect geographic distribution. Primary-care physicians who lack board certification and who encounter obstacles to specialized services are more likely to practice in areas where blacks receive their care—namely, poorer neighborhoods, as measured by the median income. Bach and his colleagues suggest that these differences play a considerable role in racial disparities in health care and health status. They make a connection between well-established facts: that physicians who are not board-certified are less likely to follow screening recommendations and more likely to manage symptoms rather than pursue diagnosis. Thus, rates of screening for breast and cervical cancer or high blood pressure are lower among black patients than white, and black patients are more likely to receive a diagnosis when their diseases are at an advanced stage.

Limited access to specialty services similarly puts black patients at a disadvantage. The Bach study is the first to examine physicians' access to specialty care and nonemergency hospital admissions in light of the race of the patients they treat. That capacities of doctors who treat black patients may account for some part of the health gap was considered in a 2002 study by researchers at the Harvard School of Public Health. The study found that physicians working for Medicare managed-care plans in which black patients were heavily enrolled provided lower-quality care to all patients. Specifically, their patients were less likely to receive the four clinical services the authors measured—mammography, eye exam for diabetics, beta-blocker after myocardial infarction, and follow-up after hospitalization for mental illness.[2]

A report in the *American Journal of Public Health* in 2000 found that blacks in a sample of almost thirty thousand patients in New York State undergoing cardiovascular surgery in 1996 had poorer access to high-quality surgeons than did whites.[3] Even among patients at the same hospital, whites were treated by better-performing surgeons, a phenomenon that may reflect some selection of patients by surgeons based on insurance coverage.[4] Donald Gemson of the Columbia University School of Public Health and colleagues showed that foreign-trained physicians and doctors not board-certified were more likely to treat black patients in New York City than to treat whites. They also found that practitioners whose caseload was more than 50 percent black or Hispanic were less likely to follow nationally recognized treatment guidelines, such as recommending mammograms or flu vaccinations for the elderly.[5] Kevin Heslin of Charles R. Drew University and his team showed a correlation between physicians' experience in treating HIV and the race of their HIV patients, with HIV-positive black patients more likely to be treated by physicians less experienced with the disease.[6]

At the Center for Studying Health System Change in Washington, D.C., J. Lee Hargraves and colleagues used the Community Tracking Study Physician Survey, a nationally representative study of American physicians, to assess their abilities to obtain medically necessary services for their patients.[7] Physicians were asked how often they could arrange referrals to specialists and inpatient admissions for their patients. According to the survey, black physicians were more likely to report difficulties admitting patients to hospitals than white physicians, and Hispanic physicians were more likely to report having a poor specialty-referral network than white physicians.

It is important to recognize that many of the physicians working in black communities are hardworking, committed individuals who earn considerably less than other doctors. As Bach's team notes, they deliver more charity care than doctors who mostly treat white patients, and derive a higher volume of their practice revenue from Medicaid, a program whose fees are notoriously low. They are often solo practitioners who scramble to make good referrals for their patients but are stymied by a dearth of well-trained colleagues and by limited access to professional networks with advanced diagnostic techniques.

While some might be willing to describe these access differentials as "discrimination" in some broad sense, the solutions to this kind of problem are substantially different from remedies premised on physician bias. Further, from a policy standpoint, resources mistakenly devoted to mitigating the problem of individual bias generally will not be available to improve access to high-quality medical care for minority individuals.

8

Patient-Side Factors Influence
Health Disparities

So far we've examined differences among doctors and hospitals serving minority populations that might account for race-related treatment differences. But what about differences in the patient populations themselves?

Self-Care

Built into the biased-doctor model is an assumption that solutions must come from providers and the system. To be sure, there is always room for greater self-awareness on the part of practitioners and for quality improvement on the part of the system, but if we fail to emphasize the role played by patients themselves, we abandon any hope of narrowing the health gap. Simply put, different racial groups have different behavioral profiles, and concentrating on the patient's side of decision-making is an essential element of improving minority health. But, again, these differences are less a characteristic of race, per se, than class.

Poorer, less-educated individuals are more likely to engage in risky behavior, such as smoking and excessive use of alcohol, and are less likely to initiate health-conscious activities, such as dieting and exercise.[1] Among African-Americans, who as a group are disproportionately poorer and less educated than whites, chronic conditions such as heart disease, stroke, lung cancer, HIV, and diabetes, whose progress can generally be arrested through self-care, represent major causes of death.[2] One-third of black women are obese, according to the Centers for Disease Control (CDC). They are nearly twice as likely as white women and more than five times as likely as Asian/ Pacific Islander women to be obese.[3]

A striking study by Ashwini Sehgal in *The Journal of the American Medical Association* reveals the importance of self-care. The team analyzed the impact of a Medicare-funded quality-improvement initiative on black-white differences in adequacy of hemodialysis, anemia, and nutritional status. They discovered that the initiative was able to equalize treatments that were simply given to the patient by medical staff, such as hemodialysis. But when it came to conditions that respond to self-care (such as anemia and other nutritional problems, which require patients to eat better or take prescribed dietary supplements regularly), the initiative was unsuccessful. It is important to recognize that failures of self-care are not signs of bias in the health care system. Poorer glycemic control among African-American patients has been documented in several cross-sectional population-based samples.[4]

David Williams of the University of Michigan and Pamela Braboy Jackson of Indiana University note that the prevalence of some diseases—such as heart disease and cancer, which are chronic—differs between blacks and whites, while that of others (such as pneumonia and flu, which are acute) does not.[5] The virtual elimination of disparities in treatment of common viral illnesses, they state, reflects several factors: widely available and simple technology, such as immunization, facilitated by Medicare and Medicaid; patient involvement that does not demand high levels of motivation, knowledge, or resources; and the fact that the intervention is applied only once. And, of course, it is motivation, knowledge, and resources that all play a vital role in decisions to exercise and to avoid certain foods, cigarettes, drugs, and excessive alcohol, to adhere to treatment regimens, and to seek treatment for medical care before illness becomes advanced.[6]

Health Literacy

Health literacy refers to the ability to understand written or spoken health information and make informed decisions on the basis of it.

According to the U.S. Department of Education, nearly half of all American adults—ninety million people—have trouble reading and thus are at risk for making poor health decisions. Forty million adults scored at the lowest of five levels, level one, on the National Adult Literacy Survey, and fifty million scored at level two.[7]

Compared to white adults, blacks were about three times as likely to score at level one in prose skills, document reading, and quantitative skills, and about 50 percent more likely to fall into level two. In practical terms, these levels correspond to having trouble finding two or more numbers on a chart and performing a calculation; coordinating several bits of information from a single document; or locating bits of information or numbers in a lengthy text. Poor understanding of the importance of monitoring and lack of ability to learn how to do it have obvious consequences for patients with medical conditions that require ongoing self-management.

Low literacy occurs disproportionately among the poor and near-poor, the elderly, those living in the South and Northeast, minorities and, of course, those with fewer years of education. Language barriers contribute to poorer asthma management among non–English-speaking Latino children compared to English-speaking Latino, white, and black children.[8] Most studies found that poor adherence to medical regimens was linked to lower literacy and levels of education. The idea that intelligence plays a role in health differentials across a population has been examined as well.[9]

Literacy has consequences for health. In 2004 the Agency for Healthcare Research and Quality reported that weak reading skills and poor comprehension were linked to higher rates of hospitalization and use of expensive (and avoidable) emergency services.[10] Poorly educated individuals less often obtained preventive services like pap smears, mammograms, immunization, and testing for sexually transmitted disease. Similarly, breastfeeding, an important boost to the neonatal immune system, was found to be less common among less literate women. In its 2004 report, *Health Literacy: A Prescription to End Confusion*, the Institute of Medicine similarly concluded that there is a higher rate of hospitalization and use of emergency services among patients with limited health literacy.[11]

A number of investigators have found African-Americans in their samples to be less well informed about procedures than white patients. For example, researchers from the Cleveland, Ohio, Veterans Affairs Medical Center approached nearly six hundred veterans over fifty years of age who had moderate or severe osteoarthritis to question their knowledge regarding hip or knee joint replacement and their views on the postoperative course for joint surgery.[12] Black patients were significantly less likely than whites to have more than high school education, to have had family or friends who had had joint replacement, or to report a good understanding of joint replacement as a form of treatment, and they had greater expectation of pain with the procedure.

Similarly, researchers at the Philadelphia Veterans Affairs Medical Center conducted a survey of over six hundred patients with pulmonary disease from three veterans hospital sites across the country. They found that more blacks than whites (61 percent versus 29 percent) maintained the folk belief that the spread of lung cancer was accelerated when the tumor was exposed to air during surgery and would oppose surgery because of this (19 percent versus 5 percent).[13] A study of patients with operable lung cancer conducted at Detroit's Henry Ford Health System found refusal of surgery by black patients over three times more common than by whites. (Both whites and blacks were offered the surgery at similar rates.)[14] When angioplasty or bypass surgery was recommended to 1,075 patients at a single tertiary care VA hospital in New York City, the black patients were significantly more reluctant to give consent than whites (15.4 percent versus 8.3 percent).[15]

Most data on health literacy reflect a given point in time—a snapshot, or cross-sectional, picture of health status and reading skill and comprehension. There have been experiments in which some patients, but not others, were randomly assigned to literacy programs, but such studies are usually short-term, use narrow process measures (asking, for instance, did knowledge increase?) rather than outcome measures (did health improve?), have small samples, and do not analyze the data by the subject's level of education.

Two major evaluations have focused on the role of education in improving clinically relevant health outcomes. One, by Dana Goldman and James Smith of RAND, examined large existing datasets of patients with HIV/AIDS and insulin-dependent diabetes. The researchers chose these conditions because although treatment regimens are complex, they are effective if followed carefully.

In their appraisal of the data from the HIV Cost and Services Utilization Study, Goldman and Smith found that 57 percent of college graduates always followed their treatment plans, while only 37 percent of high school dropouts did so. Income, insurance, and disease status did not appear to affect treatment adherence, while education level consistently mattered.[16]

The RAND authors also compared patient outcomes in the Diabetes Control and Complications Trial, a large clinical trial in which half the subjects with insulin-dependent diabetes were randomly assigned to intensive intervention.[17] They found that self-management of disease varied greatly with the patient's level of schooling; compliance, in turn, had a meaningful impact on patients' overall health status. One group of subjects in the study received treatment as usual, while the other was scheduled for more frequent clinic visits and received frequent telephone contacts. Within each group, subjects varied in their educational attainment. When results were interpreted by level of education, the least-educated were found to benefit the most—mainly because the well-educated were already doing a good job of adhering to their treatment plans. By following treatment-as-usual protocols, Goldman and Smith predicted, health outcomes of less-educated diabetics would deteriorate at a more rapid rate.

The second intervention evaluation, by Russell Rothman and colleagues at Vanderbilt University School of Medicine, also found that low-literacy patients benefited from intervention.[18] The researchers randomly assigned one group of patients with Type II diabetes who had poor glucose control to either of two conditions: usual care versus intensive, semimonthly contacts with a diabetes case coordinator. During these contacts, patients in the second group received ongoing education in identifying the symptoms of hyper- or hypoglycemia, simplified explanations with visual aids, and repeated assessment of their comprehension. After one year, the authors found that patients receiving the intensive-management program had superior outcomes. In particular, managed patients with low literacy and poor glucose control fared better than their counterparts who received only treatment as usual. (Those with high literacy had comparable outcomes irrespective of whether they were managed.) Finally, literacy level appeared to be a more powerful predictor of who would benefit from intervention management than race, income, or clinical status.

Whether low literacy is a direct cause of poor health outcomes is an intriguing question. The ability to read directions, calculate intervals between medication doses, and understand the basic physiology of one's condition and the consequences of neglect are surely useful, but as the Agency for Healthcare Research and Quality points out, poor reading ability could also be a proxy for poorer access to care, low conscientiousness, or low level of trust in medical providers. And are these variables, in turn, markers for adherence to treatment regimens?

In sum, there have been no studies to date that assess improvement in health status as a function of improved literacy, or literacy as a mediator of compliance in the context of race. It is reasonable to expect that the health differential would shrink if minorities with poor reading and comprehension skills benefited from such interventions as adoption of structured treatment plans and intensive patient monitoring, but this remains to be demonstrated.

9

Doctor-Patient Relationship

Miscommunication between doctor and patient or flawed inferences on the part of the physician are often ascribed to unappre-
ciated cultural differences. Though difficult to quantify the extent
to which these lead to differences in treatment, common sense
dictates that better doctor-patient interactions lead to better care
and thus to better health outcomes. Efforts to enhance the relationship between doctor and patient are called "cultural competence" training. Does this approach work? How does a "culturally
competent" doctor differ from a humanely sensitive one? And
should patients see doctors of their own race, or just the most
competent doctor available, regardless of race?

What Is Cultural Competence?

Cultural competence training is advanced as a remedy for miscommunication between doctors and patients of different racial or
ethnic backgrounds. Half of all medical school programs offer cultural competence teaching, according to a report in *The Journal of
the American Medical Association.*[1]

Cultural competence refers to a range of interventions. It can
include useful, practical accommodations intended to help health
providers care for unacculturated or immigrant populations—such
as translation services, or education of medical staff about local heal-
ing customs and commonly used remedies. But it can also entail
blatant racial sensitivity training. A sociologist writing in *Academic
Medicine*, for example, sees the need for such training in order to

counteract students' tendency to "deny social inequality, or . . . disadvantages experienced by Others, but not the accompanying privileges enjoyed by their own social group."[2] As promulgated by the HHS Office of Minority Health, cultural competence standards entail provision of language and "culturally appropriate" services, along with an injunction that clinical staff training should include discussion of the impact of "race and racism . . . on access to care, service utilization, quality of care, and health outcomes."[3] The standards for medical school accreditation, as put forth in 2003 by the Association of American Medical Colleges, require medical students to "learn to recognize cultural biases in themselves and others."[4]

At its most constructive, cultural competence is a variant of standard training in doctor-patient communication—a course that is required by all medical schools within the first two years of study. Joseph Betancourt, a physician at Harvard Medical School, describes an enlightened form of cultural competence that has "evolved from the making of assumptions about patients on the basis of their background to the implementation of the principles of patient-centered care, including exploration, empathy, and responsiveness to patients' needs, values, and preferences."[5]

In our view, Betancourt is simply describing the competent care that all patients, irrespective of racial or cultural identity, deserve. Consider Betancourt's description of an elderly Italian woman whose son asked the surgeon not to reveal to his mother that she had cancer because the knowledge would "kill her." The doctor explored the reason for secrecy and was able to negotiate with the son a comfortable way to inform the mother. In another scenario, a Hispanic woman suffered from hypertension that remained under poor control for two years despite various trials of antihypertensive drugs. When her doctor finally asked her about her understanding of the problem of high blood pressure, she told him that she could "feel" when her pressure was high, and that's when she took the medication. The doctor was then able to educate the patient how to take her pills correctly.

We wholly endorse the principles of cultural competence as set forth by Betancourt. What we question is the wisdom of "ghettoizing" cultural competence as a discrete didactic enterprise outside of standard doctor-patient relationship training. Indeed, these two cases were resolved using techniques that doctors should use with *any* patient—though they are especially likely to be called upon when patients are unsophisticated about health matters—but they do require time, unfortunately a scarce resource in many clinical settings. The common-sense approaches described by Betancourt transcend race and ethnicity. There was nothing particularly "Italian" or "Hispanic" about the clinical puzzles presented. In fact, some observers worry that cultural competence could deteriorate into an oversimplified paint-by-numbers affair that purports to teach students and physicians "how to treat" African-Americans, Asians, Latinos, and others.[6] Others recoil at the specter of a clinical milieu in which black patients will be assigned to black doctors, gay patients to gay doctors, and so on.[7]

There is no better way to affirm the universal principles of doctor-patient interaction than to consider the kind of pairing that happens in about one in five clinical encounters: the foreign doctor and the American patient.[8] This challenges the very premise upon which traditional cultural competence is based: the biased (white) doctor model.

In a moving essay, Alok Khorana, an Indian physician practicing in New York State, reflects on his experience caring for an elderly black man.[9] When he reaches an impasse with the family regarding transfer to hospice, Khorana worries that his previously trusting relationship with them has faltered because, perhaps, "they [were] thinking of me as, well, white."[10] He asks a nurse for help and she—a white woman—rather easily works with the family to accept hospice care. At first, Khorana is taken aback by her success, but after the nurse explains how she approaches "families we see that are struggling with this, black or white," Khorana remarks to himself, that "after all my handwringing and ruminating on race and race concordance, race was, at least in this case, a red herring."[11] In other words, the fact that Khorana was not black himself (he seemed to think that the family regarded him as "white") probably had little to do with his inability to engage the black family. Whatever the obstacle, it was not the mismatch between his race and the patient's family.

Racial Concordance and Preference

If the clinical encounter is marred by cultural misunderstandings, will disparities in treatment and outcome be reduced if doctor and patient are of the same race or ethnic background? The premise that such concordance between patient and doctor is important to the resolution of disparities has prompted calls for using race as a medical school admission criterion.[12] But what evidence exists to affirm the benefits of concordance?

First, what do we know about patients' preferences for same-race physicians? According to a 1994 Harris poll for the Commonwealth Fund, race does not play an especially large role in patients' attitudes about their doctors. When asked to cite the factors that "influence your choice of doctor," the physician's "nationality/race/ethnicity" ranked twelfth out of thirteen possible options.[13] Just 5 percent of whites and 12 percent of minorities said it was important. A greater proportion of Asians, 28 percent, rated race/ethnicity as important, probably owing to language barriers.[14] Even so, over 60 percent of white, black, and Hispanic respondents said they did not consider the doctor's ability to speak their language particularly relevant to their choice of doctor.[15]

For the entire sample of four thousand respondents, factors such as ease of getting an appointment, convenience of the office location, and the doctor's reputation were most influential, cited by about two-thirds.[16] In some cases, concordance is most likely an accident of location, as minority physicians are more likely than white physicians to reside near and disproportionately practice in minority neighborhoods.[17] When Commonwealth respondents who expressed dissatisfaction with their regular doctor were asked for details, only Asians claimed that race or ethnicity was the problem. (And the percentage was small—only 8 percent of

all Asian respondents.[18]) Among the subset of the entire sample
who said they "did not feel welcome" at their doctor's office, a
mere 2 percent of African-Americans and Hispanics and 4 percent
of Asians attributed the discomfort to racial-ethnic differences.[19]

The main complaint of almost all groups was the doctor's "failure to spend enough time with me."[20] And of those who were dis-
satisfied enough to change doctors, only 3 percent of Asians and
2 percent of blacks did so on the basis of the physician's race or
ethnicity.[21] The most common complaints were "lack of communication," "didn't like him or her," "couldn't diagnose problem,"
and "didn't trust his or her judgment."[22] Less than 1 percent of
those who said they had limited choice about where to get care
attributed that constraint to racial or ethnic discrimination.[23]

In focus groups commissioned by the Henry J. Kaiser Family
Foundation, discussions revealed that "the most common form of
discrimination described by minority consumers was not racial
[or] ethnic, rather it was discrimination based on the ability to
pay for health services."[24] A 1999 survey by the foundation
queried almost 3,900 people about their doctors. Around 85 percent of whites, African-Americans, and Latinos rated their doctors
as good or excellent.[25] Whites and blacks were about equal in
answering "yes" when asked whether their clinicians paid enough
attention to them (89 and 87 percent, respectively), though
slightly fewer Hispanic patients said so (80 percent).[26] One in five
black individuals preferred a doctor of his own race, while 12 percent did *not* want doctors of their own race.[27] Among Hispanics
polled, 28 percent wanted doctors of their own race, and 17 percent said they did not. In a much smaller survey sponsored by
Morehouse College of Medicine in Atlanta, 28 percent of the 251
African-Americans surveyed "considered it important that their
doctor be of the same ethnic group as themselves."[28]

Studies of concordance do not show consistently positive
effects of doctor-patient matching on various measures of care.[29]
Only a handful of studies have been devoted to the question of
whether patients' outcomes are better if they and their clinicians
are of the same race. Many of these studies were conducted with

psychiatric patients, and most showed that clinicians' race had a minimal impact on how black patients fared in their treatment and recovery.[30] One large study that appeared in the journal *Psychiatric Services* involved more than 1,700 homeless individuals participating in an intensive services program. Each person was randomly assigned a case manager with whom he worked closely. Over the course of a year, improvement in dimensions like the number of days a patient worked at a job, whether he had drug problems, and the number of days he spent homeless bore no relationship to whether he and the case manager were of the same race.[31] A recent study from the University of North Carolina found that physician race had little effect on the successful management of high blood pressure in elderly black and white patients. Seeing the same physician, however, was a key factor in good outcome.[32]

Other researchers have looked at the doctor-patient relationship in a different way. In one recent study, led by Lisa Cooper-Patrick of Johns Hopkins University School of Medicine and published in *The Journal of the American Medical Association*, patients gave their doctor visits a "participation score" based on the frequency with which they felt the doctor involved them in treatment decisions. Cooper-Patrick reports that black patients rated their visits as more "participatory" when their doctors were black.[33]

A closer look at the Cooper-Patrick data, however, leaves one unsure about its clinical significance. In particular, patients rated their interactions with same-race physicians (a participation score of 62.6 out of a possible 120) as barely different than interactions with different-race physicians (60.4 out of 120).[34] Using the same survey instrument, Kaplan and colleagues discovered that minority patients who saw minority doctors had *lower* scores on the questions of participation that those who saw white doctors.[35]

Evidence that race concordance between patient and physician improves care is, at best, inconsistent. One of the most effective ways to enhance the doctor-patient relationship is for doctors to spend more time with each patient. In her study, Cooper-Patrick found that the amount of time the doctor spent with the patient was linked to higher participatory ratings comparable to the ratings given by the patient when his race matched his doctor's, while Kaplan observed that the amount of time the patient spent with the doctor helped determine the participation score.[36] In the latter study, visits of less than twenty minutes were found to be too brief to involve patients in treatment decisions. In another analysis led by Kaplan, physicians who had "high-volume" practices were rated as less participatory than those who saw fewer patients but spent more time with each.[37] Given the value patients place on face-to-face time with their physician, no matter what his race, the real problem seems to be that an average primary care visit is fifteen minutes for everyone—rather than its being a few minutes shorter for black patients.[38]

Other standard features of a good doctor-patient relationship include sustaining eye-contact, minimally interrupting the patient when he is speaking, offering careful explanations of treatments and options, encouraging patients to ask questions, and so on. The physician must be alert to the idea that a patient's culture might interfere with the interview or willingness to accept care (for instance, some patients of Asian descent may be reluctant to make eye-contact), but unless he regularly serves patients of particular backgrounds, the physician cannot be expected to know idiosyncrasies of multiple groups.

Furthermore, sex, age, social class, and education make a big difference in concordance of doctor and patient medical knowledge. Take the example of black pediatrician Lynn Smitherman, who wrote a paper in *Pediatrics* entitled, "Use of Folk Remedies Among Children in an Urban Black Community: Remedies for Fever, Colic and Teething."[39] On a radio show she explained that she wrote the paper because she hadn't heard of any of the remedies—her mother and grandmother did not use any with her when she was a child—and assumed that many of her colleagues might not be familiar with them either. Similarly, many black trainees or physicians may not be any more aware of certain folk beliefs than whites—for example, the notions that air causes a cancer to spread, that the devil can cause a person to get cancer, or that chiropractic is an effective treatment for breast cancer.[40] Clearly, not all black Americans share the same cultural experiences.

Finally, the patient has a role in facilitating his care. The doctor can encourage patients who are less educated, unfamiliar with clinical encounters, or reticent during visits to bring advocates or family members with them.[41] Educational modules that prepare and coach patients to ask questions and present information about themselves to their doctors are promising where implemented.[42]

Conclusion

To return to the question we posed at the beginning—would a white and black patient arriving at the emergency room receive the same care?—we see that the question itself (at least as it is commonly understood) is flawed. The question presumes that black and white patients frequent the same health-care services, carry the same insurance coverage, and have identical health conditions—yet the data reveal that often they do not.

The most obvious and influential causes of these disparities reside in the differing health resources available to blacks and whites, including the quality of the physicians who treat them. These features place the emphasis on aspects of the health-care system in generating race-related differentials in treatment and far less so on clinically unjustifiable differences in treatment of white and minority patients by a given physician.

Meanwhile, true physician "bias" is very difficult to measure and define (since rational inferences are not the same as genuine prejudice). The Institute of Medicine panel might well have come to that conclusion itself had Congress directed it to evaluate the relative contributions of geographic, demographic, social, and economic factors in explaining discrepancies in care and outcomes. With that charge, the panel might well have come to a similar conclusion about the contribution of bias and the dubious value of emphasizing its role in maintaining the care gap and trying to combat it.

But if physicians cannot fairly be accused of bias, does this just shift the charge of bias to the health-care system? In other words, do black patients receive poorer care because they are black or because they have disproportionately lower incomes and social capital (for example, less capacity for negotiating complex systems) than whites—and are thus disproportionately mired in systems that are underfinanced?

The most recent report from the Agency for Healthcare Research and Quality suggests this is so. It examines, separately, quality by race and quality by income.[1] It says that "remote rural populations" receive poor care, and "many racial and ethnic minorities and persons of lower socioeconomic positions" receive suboptimal care.[2] But a better test of the class-trumps-race hypothesis would be to compare the quality of care received by poor whites clustered in a particular geographic area, for example, Appalachian populations, to that received by poor blacks who are clustered, for example, in southeast Washington, D.C. If, after accounting for regional differences in practice or in health-care financing, comparable (and suboptimal) care were demonstrated, this would provide powerful support for the idea that systems serving poor people, irrespective of race, provide lower-quality care. Until such data are published— surprisingly we could find no reports on care of low-income whites versus low-income minorities—the allegation of racial bias in the system is unsupported.[3]

Fortunately, policymakers are attuned to the quality problem and are grappling with it on several fronts, including the promotion and spread of information technology, performance enhancement of medical systems, outcome-based reimbursement to providers, and provider incentives (including malpractice reform, tax breaks, and assertion of market mechanisms that, among other things, reward physicians for the time they spend with patients).[4] They also recognize that low-income patients benefit from a strong safety net provided by the federally funded community health-care system (guaranteeing a usual source of care); grassroots outreach through black churches, social clubs, and worksites; patient "navigators" to help negotiate the system; language services; and efforts to get more good doctors into distressed neighborhoods.[5] Seemingly simple innovations, such as clinic night hours, could be a great boon to patients with hourly-wage employment who risk a loss of income, or even their jobs, by taking time off from work for doctors' appointments.

Much has been made of the need for greater sensitivity in the doctor-patient relationship.[6] Common sense dictates that patients benefit when they trust their physicians and interact with them productively. But the remedies for unsatisfactory doctor-patient relationships do not reside in racial sensitivity training for health-care professionals, or the specter of Title VI litigation.

Rather, the true remedies to these problems would be fostered by the opportunity for the patient to see the same physician on each visit with ample time to discuss problems, and to be seen by a physician who, as Betancourt put it, engages in "exploration, empathy, and responsiveness to patients' needs, values, and preferences."

Ultimately, improvement in the quality of care and self-care would elevate the status of minority health appreciably. But the greater public-health good would be served by applying these goals to all underserved people, rather than focusing on minorities. By focusing on those with the worst health, as Stephen Isaacs and Steven Schroeder have pointed out, the targets of intervention will still turn out to be poor minority groups, but they will include lower-class whites as well.[7] For example, establishing screening (for cancer, diabetes, or hypertension) or wellness-education programs in benighted areas such as southeast Washington, D.C., or the Watts neighborhood of Los Angeles would benefit all residents and would shrink overall racial differentials in health outcome because they would disproportionately target minorities.

Targeting the underserved also changes the metric by which success is measured. That is, instead of trying to equalize the use of procedures and treatments in minorities versus whites, the goal should be high-quality care for everyone. As Baicker and Chandra point out, this makes sense for interventions that are considered effective preventive care, such as mammograms for women over fifty and eye exams for diabetics.[8] Indeed, this is exactly what Trivedi's study showed. His data, collected before deliberate efforts to reduce gaps in preventive care had begun, showed that quality improvement in general helped black patients disproportionately.[9] In contrast, for costly procedures whose administration depends partly on patient preference and whose "correct" rate of use is unknown, the goal should be for each patient in need to be well-informed and have choices of high-quality treatment.

Perhaps one of the most important factors in health disparities—self-care—does not depend much on health systems, except, perhaps, as vehicles for education. As Isaacs and Schroeder point out, medical-care failures have been estimated to account for only about 10–15 percent of premature deaths.[10] It is behaviors such as smoking, excessive alcohol use, unhealthy dietary patterns, and lack of exercise that figure so prominently in the development and course of chronic disease. In this arena, too, the influence of class outstrips race. Along these lines, Avis Thomas of the University of Minnesota and colleagues have found that after adjustment for income and risk factors such as blood pressure, cholesterol, and smoking, the rate of coronary heart disease in blacks and whites becomes equal.[11]

Words such as "prejudice," "bias," and "discrimination" are charged and divisive. Civil rights advocates talk about the lingering shadow cast by troubled race relations on the health-care system. Yet, paradoxically, health campaigns that seek to educate about alleged bias of physicians will only inflame the mistrust that some minority patients already harbor. Concentrating on improving the health of all underserved Americans is the most fair and efficient public health agenda.

Notes

Introduction

1. Harold P. Freeman, "Race, Poverty, and Cancer: Comprehensive Care for All" (speech, conference sponsored by the Center For Mind-Body Medicine, National Institutes of Health's Office of Alternative Medicine (OAM), and the University of Texas–Houston Health Science Center Medical School of Nursing, Arlington, Va., January 12, 1998), http://www.cmbm.org/conferences/ccc98/transcripts/Freeman.doc (accessed November 7, 2005).

2. U.S. Department of Health and Human Services, *Report of the Secretary's Task Force on Black and Minority Health* (Washington, D.C., U.S. Government Printing Office), August 1985.

3. Jack Geiger and Gretchen Borchelt, "Racial and Ethnic Disparities in US Health Care," *Lancet* 362 (2003): 1674; Talmudge King and Margaret Wheeler, "Inequality in Health Care: Unjust, Inhumane, and Unattended," *Annals of Internal Medicine* 141, no. 10 (2004): 815–17.

4. Brian D. Smedley, Adrienne Y. Stith, and Alan R. Nelson, eds., *Unequal Treatment: Confronting Racial and Ethnic Disparities in Health Care* (Washington, D.C.: National Academy of Sciences, 2002)

5. *Newsday*, "Color-Blind Care . . . Is Not What Minorities Are Getting from U.S. Physicians. It's Time for That to Change," March 2002, A28; Michael Lasalandra, "Fed Report Cites 'Prejudice' in White, Minority Health Care Gap," *Boston Herald*, March 21, 2002, 012; *St. Louis Post-Dispatch* (Missouri), "Separate and Unequal," March 24, 2002, B2.

6. Lucille Perez, statement at IOM press conference, March 19, 2002, http://www.nmanet.org/ pr_032502.htm (accessed May 22, 2005).

7. Richard Epstein, "Disparities and Discrimination in Health Care Coverage: A Critique of the Institute of Medicine Study," Working Paper No. 208, John M. Olin Center for Law and Economics, University of Chicago, 2004, 29.

8. David Barton Smith, "Racial and Ethnic Health Disparities and the Unfinished Civil Rights Agenda," *Health Affairs* 24, no. 2 (2005): 323.

9. Some of these data were published after the 2002 release of the IOM report but, as we explain below, the congressional mandate to the panel sent it in a particular direction that narrowed its focus. A recent paper that sought to update the literature following the IOM report reviewed only one study that focused on geography as the independent variable; see Judith A. Long and others, "Update on the Health Disparities Literature," *Annals of Internal Medicine* 141, no. 10 (2004): 805–12.

10. For a review of studies see Sally Satel and Jonathan Klick, "The Institute of Medicine Report: Too Quick to Diagnose Bias," *Perspectives in Biology and Medicine* 48, no. 1. supp. (2004): S15–S25.

11. Berlin J. Schulman and others, "The Effect of Race and Sex on Physicians' Recommendations for Cardiac Catheterization," *New England Journal of Medicine* 340, no. 8 (1999): 618–26. In this study, doctors rated whites as more likely to sue.

12. Daniel Kessler and Mark McClellan, "Do Doctors Practice Defensive Medicine?" *The Quarterly Journal of Economics* 111, no. 2 (May 1996): 353–90.

13. Katherine Baicker and others, "Who You Are and Where You Live: How Race and Geography Affect the Treatment of Medicare Beneficiaries," *Health Affairs*, web exclusive, October 7, 2004, http://content.health affairs.org/cgi/content/abstract/hlthaff.var.33v1 (accessed August 29, 2005).

14. June Eichner and Bruce C. Vladeck, "Medicare as a Catalyst for Reducing Health Disparities," *Health Affairs* 24, no. 2 (2005): 365–75.

15. Amal N. Trivedi and others, "Trends in Quality of Care and Racial Disparities for Enrollees in Medicare Managed Care," *New England Journal of Medicine* 353, no. 7 (2005): 43–51.

16. David Mechanic, "Policy Challenges in Addressing Racial Disparities and Improving Population Health," *Health Affairs* 24, no. 2 (2005): 336.

17. Ibid.

18. Stephen L. Isaacs and Steven A. Schroeder, "Class—The Ignored Determinant of the Nation's Health," *New England Journal of Medicine* 351, no. 11 (2004): 1137–42; Ichiro Kawachi, Norman Daniels, and Dean E. Robinson, "Health Disparities by Race and Class: Why Both Matter," *Health Affairs* 24, no. 2 (2005): 336.

19. National Center for Health Statistics, *Health, United States, 1998, with Socioeconomic Status and Health Chartbook* (Hyattsville, Md.: NCHS).

20. David R. Williams and Chiquita Collins, "U.S. Socioeconomic and Racial Differences in Health Patterns and Explanations," *Annual Review of Sociology* 21 (1995): 349–86; George Davey Smith and others, "1998 Mortality Differences Between Black and White Men in the USA:

Contribution of Income and Other Risk Factors Among Men Screened for the MRFIT," *Lancet* 351 (1998): 934–39.

21. Sara Rosenbaum and Joel B. Teitelbaum, "Civil Rights Enforcement in the Modern Health Care System: Reinvigorating the Role of the Federal Government in the Aftermath of *Alexander v. Sandoval*," *Yale Journal of Health Policy, Law, and Ethics* 3, no. 2 (2003): 215–52; Michael Shin, "Redressing Wounds: Finding a Legal Framework to Remedy Racial Disparities in Medical Care," *California Law Review* 90 (2002): 2047–2100.

Chapter 1

1. U.S. Department of Health and Human Services, Agency for Healthcare Research and Quality, "National Healthcare Disparities Report 2003" (Rockville, Md.: U.S. Department of Health and Human Services, 2003) http://www.qualitytools.ahrq.gov/disparitiesreport/archive/2003/download/download_report.aspx (accessed November 23, 2005).

2. Olivia Carter-Pokras and Claudia Baquet, "What is a 'Health Disparity?'" *Public Health Reports* 117 (2002): 427.

3. M. Gregg Bloche, "Health Care Disparities—Science, Politics, and Race," *New England Journal of Medicine* 350, no. 15 (2004): 1568–70.

4. Consortium of Social Science Associations, "House Senate Members Protest Changes To Scientific Report On Health Disparities," *COSSA: Washington Update* 23, no. 2 (January 26, 2004), http://www.cossa.org/volume23/23.2.htm (accessed June 14, 2005).

5. *Black Issues in Higher Education*, "Health Disparities Report at Center of Controversy; Department Altered Scientists' Conclusions to Fit 'Political Goals,' Lawmakers Say," February 12, 2004.

6. Congressional Black Caucus Foundation, "National Medical Association Appalled Over Distorted HHS Disparities Report," February 10, 2004, http://www.cbcfhealth.org/content/contentID/2419 (accessed May 4, 2005).

7. Leonard S. Rubenstein and Gretchen Borchelt, "Administration's Reality Gap on Health Disparities," Center for American Progress, September 20, 2004, http://www.americanprogress.org (accessed May 29, 2005).

8. Smedley and others, *Unequal Treatment*, 1.

9. Louis Sullivan, "From the Secretary of Health and Human Services," *The Journal of the American Medical Association* 266, no. 19 (1991): 2674.

10. Curtis L. Taylor, "The Health Divide/Mistakes in the Past, Fears in the Present/Wary of System, Many Blacks Reluctant to Seek Timely Care," *Newsday*, December 4, 1998.

11. U.S.Commission on Civil Rights. "The Health Care Challenge: Acknowledging Disparity, Confronting Discrimination and Ensuring

Equality," vol. 2, "The Role of Federal Civil Rights Enforcement Efforts" (September 1999), 14.

12. Edward M. Kennedy, "The Role of the Federal Government in Eliminating Health Disparities," *Health Affairs* 24, no. 2 (2005): 457.

13. Marian Wright Edelman, remarks to the class of 2005, Colgate University, May 16, 2005, http://www.colgate.edu/DesktopDefault1 .aspx?tabid=730&pgID=6013&nwID=3762 (accessed May 24, 2005).

14. Jose J. Escarce, "How Does Race Matter, Anyway?" *Health Services Research* 40, no. 1 (2005): 1–7.

15. *Healthcare Equality and Accountability Act of 2003*, 108th Cong., 1st sess. *Congressional Record* S3967–68 (November 6, 2003): S 1833.

16. American Medical Association, "Improving Immunization: Addressing Racial and Ethnic Populations," Roadmaps for Clinical Practice Series, June 2005, http://www.ama-assn.org/ama/pub/category/9958.html (accessed July 19, 2005).

17. American Public Health Association, "Research and Intervention on Racism as a Fundamental Cause of Ethnic Disparities in Health," http://www.apha.org/legislative/policy/policysearch/index.cfm?fuseaction= view&id=246 (accessed January 20, 2005).

18. U.S. Department of Health and Human Services, National Institutes of Health, "The Effect of Racial and Ethnic Discrimination/Bias on Health Care Delivery," program announcement no. PA-05-006, expiration date January 3, 2008, http://www.ama-assn.org/ama/pub/category/9958.html (accessed August 31, 2005).

19. Jordan J. Cohen, "The Consequences of Premature Abandonment of Affirmative Action in Medical School Admissions," *The Journal of the American Medical Association* 289, no. 9 (2003): 1143–49; Neil Calman, "Out of the Shadows: A White Doctor Wrestles with Racial Prejudice," *Health Affairs* 19, no. 1 (2000): 170–74.

20. Shawn Rhea, "Cultural Training Required from Doctors," *Camden Courier Post*, March 24, 2005, http://www.courierpostonline.com/news/ southjersey/m032405a.htm (accessed July 1, 2005).

21. Ana I. Balsa and Thomas G. McGuire, "Prejudice, Clinical Uncertainty and Stereotyping as Sources of Health Disparities," *Journal of Health Economics* 22, no. 1 (2003): 89–116.

22. Olivia Carter-Pokras and Claudia Baquet, "What is a 'Health Disparity'?"; Saif Rathore and Harlan Krumholz, "Differences, Disparities, and Biases: Clarifying Racial Variations in Health Care Use," *Annals of Internal Medicine* 141, no. 8 (2004): 635–38.

23. National Institutes of Health, "Addressing Health Disparities: The NIH Program in Action," 2004, http://healthdisparities.nih.gov/whatare .html (accessed February 4, 2005).

24. National Center on Minority Health and Health Disparities, "Mission Statement," http://ncmhd.nih.gov/about_ncmhd/mission.asp (accessed May 4, 2005).

25. National Institutes of Health, "Strategic Research Plan and Budget to Reduce and Ultimately Eliminate Health Disparities," vol. 1, http://ncmhd.nih.gov/our_programs/strategic/pubs/VolumeI_031003EDrev.pdf (accessed February 10, 2005).

26. U.S. Department of Health and Human Services, *Healthy People 2010: Understanding and Improving Health* (Washington, D.C.: U.S. Government Printing Office, 2000).

27. *Minority Health and Health Disparity Research and Education Act of 2000*, Public Law 106-525, 106th Cong., 2nd sess. (November 22, 2000).

28. Smedley and others, *Unequal Treatment*, 4.

29. Thomas LaVeist, *Minority Populations and Health: An Introduction to Health Disparities in the United States* (San Francisco, Calif.: Jossey-Bass, 2005), 109.

30. Jordan J. Cohen, "Disparities in Health Care: An Overview," *Academic Emergency Medicine* 10, no. 11 (2003): 1155–60; Geiger and Borchelt, "Racial and Ethnic Disparities in US Health Care"; Carol J. Rowland Hogue, "Toward a Systemic Approach to Understanding—and Ultimately Eliminating—African American Women's Health Disparities," *Women's Health* 12, no. 5 (2002): 225–30; L. Sullivan and others, *Missing Persons: Minorities in the Health Professions. A Report of the Sullivan Commission on Diversity in the Healthcare Workforce* (Atlanta, Georgia, 2004), http://admissions.duhs.duke.edu/sullivancommission/index.cfm, accessed November 21, 2005.

Chapter 2

1. Adewale Troutman, interview by Ray Suarez, "Unequal Treatment," *NewsHour with Jim Lehrer*, PBS, March 9, 2005.

2. Smedley and others, *Unequal Treatment*, 3.

3. Peter Bach and others, "Patient Demographic and Socioeconomic Characteristics in the SEER-Medicare Database Applications and Limitations," *Medical Care* 40, no. 8, (2002): IV-19–IV-25; Janice M. Barnhart, Sylvia Wassertheil-Smoller, and E. Scott Monrad, "Clinical and Nonclinical Correlates of Racial and Ethnic Differences in Recommendation Patterns for Coronary Revascularization," *Clinical Cardiology* 23, no. 8 (2002): 580–86; Alain G. Bertoni and others, "Racial and Ethnic Disparities in Cardiac Catheterization from Acute Myocardial Infarction in the United States 1995–2001," *Journal of the National Medical Association* 97, no. 3 (2005): 317–23.

4. Smedley and others, *Unequal Treatment*, 50.

5. Reginald Peniston and others, "Severity of Coronary Artery Disease in Black and White Male Veterans and Likelihood of Revascularization," *American Heart Journal* 139, no. 5 (2000): 840–47.

6. Donald M. Berwick, "Disseminating Innovations in Health Care," *The Journal of the American Medical Association* 289 (2003): 1969–75; Baicker and others, "Who You Are and Where You Live"; Saif S. Rathore and others, "Regional Variations in Racial Differences in the Treatment of Elderly Patients Hospitalized with Acute Myocardial Infarction," *American Journal of Medicine* 117, no. 11 (2004): 811–22; Peter W. Groeneveld, Paul A. Heidenreich, and Alan M. Garber, "Trends in Implantable Cardioverter-Defibrillator Racial Disparity," *Journal of the American College of Cardiology* 45, no. 1 (2005): 72–78; Jonathan S. Skinner and others, "Racial, Ethnic and Geographical Disparities in Rates of Knee Arthroplasty Among Medicare Recipients," *New England Journal of Medicine* 349, no. 14 (2003): 1350–59; Amitabh Chandra and Jonathan S. Skinner, "Geography and Racial Health Disparities," NBER Working Paper 9513 (Washington D.C.: National Bureau of Economic Research, Inc., 2003); Jing Fang and Michael H. Alderman, "Is Geography Destiny for Patients in New York with Myocardial Infarction?" *American Journal of Medicine* 115, no. 6 (2003): 452–53.

7. Baicker and others, "Who You Are and Where You Live"; Rathore and others, "Regional Variations in Racial Differences in the Treatment of Elderly Patients"; Groeneveld and others, "Trends in Implantable Cardioverter-Defibrillator Racial Disparity"; Skinner and others, "Racial, Ethnic and Geographical Disparities in Rates of Knee Arthroplasty"; Chandra and Skinner, "Geography and Racial Health Disparities"; Fang and Alderman, "Is Geography Destiny?"

8. Katherine Baicker and others, "Who You Are and Where You Live."

9. Personal communication with "Kathy A.," Johns Hopkins nurse practitioner, 2003.

10. Gary C. Curhan, "A 44 year old woman with kidney stones," *The Journal of the American Medical Association* 293, no. 9 (2005): 1110.

11. Robert Rubin, MD (professor of medicine, Georgetown University School of Medicine), personal communication, March 10, 2005.

12. Michael Marmot, *The Status Syndrome: How Social Standing Affects Our Health and Longevity* (London: Bloomsbury Publishing, 2005).

13. Schulman and others, "The Effect of Race and Sex on Physicians' Recommendations for Cardiac Catheterization."

14. Thomas H. Maugh II, "Study Overstated Racism, Heart Disease Link, Journal Says," *Los Angeles Times,* July 26, 1999; "Cardiac Testing: Study Finds Women, Blacks Are Being Shortchanged," *Chicago Tribune*, March 18, 1999.

15. Lisa M. Schwartz, Steven Woloshin, and H. Gilbert Welch, "Misunderstandings about the Effect of Race and Sex on Physicians' Referrals for Cardiac Catheterization," *New England Journal of Medicine* 341, no. 4 (1999): 279–83.

16. Ibid., 282.

17. Ted Koppel, *Nightline*, February 24, 1999.

18. Jersey Chen and others, "Racial Differences in the Use of Cardiac Catheterization After Acute Myocardial Infarction," *New England Journal of Medicine* 344, no. 19 (2001): 1443–49.

19. Donald A. Barr, "Racial Differences in the Use of Cardiac Catheterization," *New England Journal of Medicine* 345, no. 11 (2001): 839.

20. Chen and others, "Racial Differences in the Use of Cardiac Catheterization After Acute Myocardial Infarction."

21. Padma Kaul and others, "Influence of Racial Disparities in Procedure Use on Functional Status Outcomes Among Patients with Coronary Artery Disease," *Circulation* 111 (2005):1284–90. The following studies have documented more complications following surgery for blacks than for whites: Edward L. Hannan and others, "Predictors of Readmission for Complications of Coronary Artery Bypass Graft Surgery," *Journal of the American Medical Association* 290 (2003): 773–80; Nizar N. Mahomed and others, "Rates and Outcomes of Primary and Revision Total Hip Replacement in the United States Medicare Population," *The Journal of Bone and Joint Surgery (American)* 85-A, no. 1 (2003): 27–32; Jennifer A. Heller and others, "Two Decades of Abdominal Aortic Aneurysm Repair: Have We Made Any Progress?" *Journal of Vascular Surgery* 32, no. 6 (2000): 1091–1100; Donald A. Morris and others, "Risk Factors for Early Filtration Failure Requiring Suture Release after Primary Glaucoma Triple Procedure with Adjunctive Mitomycin," *Archives of Ophthalmology* 117, no. 9 (1999): 1149–54.

22. Joseph P. Newhouse, *Free For All: Lessons from the RAND Health Insurance Experiment* (Cambridge, Mass.: Harvard University Press, 1996).

23. Henry J. Kaiser Family Foundation, "Racial/Ethnic Differences in Cardiac Care: The Weight of the Evidence," summary report, October 2002, appendix A. The following studies were among those listed in appendix A with mortality outcome data: John G. Canto and others, "Presenting Characteristics, Treatment Patterns, and Clinical Outcomes Of Non-Black Minorities in the National Registry of Myocardial Infarction," *American Journal of Cardiology* 82, no. 9 (1998): 1013–18; Chen and others, "Racial Differences in the Use of Cardiac Catheterization After Acute Myocardial Infarction"; Joseph Conigliaro and others, "Understanding Racial Variation in the Use of Coronary Revascularization Procedures: The

Role of Clinical Factors," *Archives of Internal Medicine* 160, no. 9 (2000): 1329–35; Marian E. Gornick and others, "Effects of Race and Income on Mortality and the Use of Services among Medicare Beneficiaries," *New England Journal of Medicine* 335, no. 11 (1996): 791–99; Patrice M. Gregory and others, "Impact of Availability of Hospital-Based Invasive Cardiac Services on Racial Differences in the Use of these Services," *American Heart Journal* 138, no. 3, pt. 1 (1999): 507–17; Charles Maynard and others, "Long-Term Implications of Racial Differences in the Use of Revascularization Procedures (The Myocardial Infarction Triage and Intervention Registry)," *American Heart Journal* 133, no. 6 (1997): 656–62; Judith Mickelson, Cynthia M. Blum, and Jane M. Geraci, "Acute Myocardial Infarction: Clinical Characteristics, Management and Outcome in a Metropolitan Veterans Affairs Medical Center Teaching Hospital," *Journal of the American College of Cardiology* 29, no. 5 (1999): 915–25; Albert Oberman and Gary Cutter, "Issues in the Natural History and Treatment of Coronary Heart Disease in Black Populations: Surgical Treatment," *American Heart Journal* 108, no. 3, pt. 2 (1984): 688–94; Peniston and others, "Severity of Coronary Artery Disease in Black and White Male Veterans"; Eric D. Peterson, "Racial Variation in Cardiac Procedure Use and Survival Following Acute Myocardial Infarction in the Department of Veterans Affairs," *The Journal of the American Medical Association* 271, no. 15 (1994): 1175–80; Steven Udvarhelyi and others, "Acute Myocardial Infarction in the Medicare Population: Process of Care and Clinical Outcomes," *The Journal of the American Medical Association* 268, no.18 (1992): 2530–36. See also Peter H. Stone and others, "Influence of Race, Sex and Age on Management of Unstable Angina and Non-Q-Wave Myocardial Infarction: The TIMI III Registry," *The Journal of the American Medical Association* 275, no. 14 (1996): 1104–12, which showed no differences in mortality or MI at six weeks post–cardiac procedure.

24. Amber Barnato and others, "Hospital-Level Racial Disparities in Acute Myocardial Infarction Treatment and Outcomes," *Medical Care* 43 (2005): 308–19.

25. Viola Vaccarino and others, "Sex and Racial Differences in the Management of Acute Myocardial Infarction, 1994 through 2002," *New England Journal of Medicine* 353, no. 7 (2005): 671–82.

26. Eric C. Schneider and others, "Racial Differences in Cardiac Revascularization Rates: Does 'Overuse' Explain Higher Rates among White Patients?" *Annals of Internal Medicine* 135, no. 5 (2001): 328–37.

27. J. E. Wennberg, E. S. Fisher, and J. S. Skinner, "Geography and the Debate over Medicare Reform," *Health Affairs*, supplemental web exclusive, content.healthaffairs.org/cgi/content/abstract/hlthaff.w2.96v1 (accessed July 9, 2005); R. J. De Winter and others, "Early Invasive Versus Selectively

Invasive Management for Acute Coronary Syndromes," *New England Journal Medicine* 353, no. 11 (2005): 1095–1104.

28. Jonathan Skinner and others, "Mortality After Acute Myocardial Infarction in Hospitals that Disproportionately Treat African Americans," *Circulation* 112 (2005): 2634–41.

29. Marc Sabatine and others, "Influence of Race on Death and Ischemic Complications in Patients with Non-ST Elevation Acute Coronary Syndromes Despite Modern, Protocol-Guided Treatment," *Circulation* 111 (2005): 1217–24.

30. Ibid., 1223.

31. Janice M. Barnhart, Jing J. Fang, and Michael H. Alderman, "Differential Use of Coronary Revascularization and Hospital Mortality Following Acute Myocardial Infarction," *Archives of Internal Medicine* 163, no. 4 (2003): 461–66.

32. Jason A. Dominitz and others, "Race, Treatment, and Survival among Colorectal Carcinoma Patients in an Equal-Access Medical System," *Cancer* 82, no. 12 (1998): 2312–20; Allen J. Taylor, Gregg S. Meyer, and Robert W. Morse, "Can Characteristics of a Health Care System Mitigate Ethnic Bias in Access to Cardiovascular Procedures? Experience from the Military Health Services System," *Journal of the American College of Cardiology* 30, no. 4 (1997): 901–7. See also Paul D. Stein and others, "Venous Thromboembolic Disease: Comparison of the Diagnostic Process in Blacks and Whites," *Archives of Internal Medicine* 163, no. 15 (2003): 1843–48. This national hospital discharge survey found no difference by race in terms of venous ultrasound, contrast venography, radioisotope lung scan, or duration of hospital stay; at the same time, age-adjusted rates of deep venous thrombosis (DVT) and pulmonary embolus (PE) were the same in blacks and whites.

33. Eugene Z. Oddone and others, "Carotid Endarterectomy and Race: Do Clinical Indications and Patient Preferences Account for Differences?" *Stroke* 33, no. 12 (2002): 2936; Charles Bennett and others, "Racial Differences in Care Among Hospitalized Patients with Pneumocystis Carinii, Pneumonia in Chicago, New York, Los Angeles, Miami, and Raleigh-Durham," *Archives of Internal Medicine* 155, no. 15 (1995): 1586–92; Larry B. Goldstein and others, "Veterans Administration Acute Stroke (VASt) Study," *Stroke* 34, no. 4 (2003): 999; Kathleen A. McGinnis and others, "Understanding Racial Disparities in HIV Using Data from the Veterans Aging Cohort 3-Site Study and VA Administrative Data," *American Journal of Public Health* 93, no. 10 (2003): 1728–33; Andrea D. Gurmankin, Daniel Polsky, and Kevin G. Volpp, "Accounting for Apparent 'Reverse' Racial Disparities in Department of Veterans Affairs (VA)-Based Medical Care: Influence of Out-of-VA Care," *American Journal of Public Health* 94,

no. 12 (2004): 2076–78; Wallace Akerley and others, "Racial Comparison of Outcomes of Male Department of Veterans Affairs Patients With Lung and Colon Cancer," *Archives of Internal Medicine* 153, no. 14 (1993): 1681–88; Peniston and others, "Severity of Coronary Artery Disease in Black and White Male Veterans."

34. Laura A. Petersen and others, "Impact of Race on Cardiac Care and Outcomes in Veterans with Acute Myocardial Infarction," *Medical Care* 40, supp. 1 (2002): 186–96; Anita Deswal and others, "Impact of Race on Health Care Utilization and Outcomes in Veterans with Congestive Heart Failure," *Journal of the American College of Cardiology* 43, no. 5 (2004): 778–84; Vincent L. Freeman and others, "Determinants of Mortality Following a Diagnosis of Prostate Cancer in Veterans Affairs and Private Sector Health Care Systems," *American Journal of Public Health* 93, no. 10 (2003): 1706–12; Ashish K. Jha and others, "Racial Differences in Mortality Among Men Hospitalized in the Veterans Affairs Health Care System," *The Journal of the American Medical Association* 285, no. 3 (2001): 297–303; Bennett and others, "Racial Differences in Care Among Hospitalized Patients with Pneumocystis Carinii"; Goldstein and others, "Veterans Administration Acute Stroke (VASt) Study"; Akerley and others, "Racial Comparison of Outcomes of Male Department of Veterans Affairs Patients With Lung and Colon Cancer."

35. James S. Rawlings and Louis W. Sullivan, "Race- and Rank-Specific Infant Mortality in a U.S. Military Population," *American Journal of Diseases of Children* 146, no. 3 (1992): 313–16; John P. Kluger, Frederick A. Connell, and Charles E. Henley, "Lack of Difference in Neonatal Mortality Between Blacks and Whites Served by the Same Medical Care System," *Journal of Family Practice* 30, no. 3 (1990): 281–88.

36. Nancy Kressin and others, "Racial Differences in Health-Related Beliefs, Attitudes, and Experiences of VA Cardiac Patients: Scale Development and Application," *Medical Care* 40, no. 1, suppl. (2002): 172–85.

Chapter 3

1. Gordon W. Allport, *The Nature of Prejudice* (Garden City, N.Y.: Doubleday, 1954).

2. Rathore and Krumholz, "Differences, Disparities, and Biases."

3. Ana I. Balsa, Thomas G. McGuire, and Lisa S. Meredith, "Testing for Statistical Discrimination in Health Care," *Health Services Research* 40, no. 1 (2005): 209–34.

4. Diana J. Burgess, Steven S. Fu, and Michelle van Ryn, "Why Do Providers Contribute to Disparities and What Can Be Done About It?" *Journal of General Internal Medicine* 19, no. 11 (2004): 1154–59; Michelle van Ryn and Steven S. Fu, "Paved with Good Intentions: Do Public Health and Human

Service Providers Contribute to Racial/Ethnic Disparities in Health?" *American Journal of Public Health* 93, no. 2 (2003): 248–55; Michelle van Ryn and Jane Burke, "The Effect of Patient Race and Socio-Economic Status on Physicians' Perceptions of Patients," *Social Science Medicine* 50, no. 6 (2000): 813–28.

5. Calman, "Out of the Shadows."

Chapter 4

1. John E. Wennberg, "The Quality of Medical Care in the United States: A Report on the Medicare Program," in John E. Wennberg and M. M. Cooper, eds., *The Dartmouth Atlas of Health Care 1999* (Hanover, N.H.: Health Forum Inc., 1999).

2. Chandra and Skinner, "Geography and Racial Health Disparities."

3. Ichiro Kawachi and Lisa Berkman, eds., *Neighborhoods and Health* (New York: Oxford University Press, 2003).

4. Katherine Baicker, Amitabh Chandra, and Jonathan S. Skinner, "Geographic Variation in Health Care and the Problem of Measuring Racial Disparities," *Perspectives in Biology and Medicine* 48, no. 1, supp. (2005): S42–53. In this paper the authors conclude that 56 percent of the differential exists between regions, and 44 percent resides within regions. When two important within-region phenomena are accounted for—the fact that blacks and whites are seen at different hospitals and that, within hospitals, different physicians often treat them—researchers can estimate the extent of the treatment gap, if any, with better accuracy.

5. Baicker and others, "Geographic Variation in Health Care."

6. Angus Deaton and Darren Lubotsky, "Mortality, Inequality and Race in American Cities and States," *Social Science Medicine* 56, no. 6 (2003): 1139–53; Alberto Alesina, Reza Baqir, and William Easterly, "Public Goods and Ethnic Divisions," Policy Research Working Paper Series 2108 (Washington, D.C.: The World Bank, 1999).

7. Skinner and others, "Mortality After Acute Myocardial Infarction."

8. Barnato and others, "Hospital-Level Racial Disparities."

9. Leo Morales and others, "Mortality Among Very Low Birthweight Infants in Hospitals Serving Minority Populations," *American Journal of Public Health* 95 (2005): 2206–12

Chapter 5

1. John D. Birkmeyer and others, "Hospital Volume and Surgical Mortality in the United States," *New England Journal of Medicine* 346, no. 15 (2003): 1128–37.

2. Elizabeth H. Bradley and others, "Racial and Ethnic Differences in Time to Acute Reperfusion Therapy for Patients Hospitalized With Myocardial Infarction," *The Journal of the American Medical Association* 292, no. 13 (2004): 1571.

3. Lucian L. Leape and others, "Underuse of Cardiac Procedures: Do Women, Ethnic Minorities, and the Uninsured Fail to Receive Needed Vascularization?" *Annals of Internal Medicine* 130, no. 3 (1999): 864–80.

4. Kevin Fiscella and others, "Racial Disparity in Surgical Complications in New York State," *Annals of Surgery* 242 (2005): 151–55.

5. Jan Blustein and Beth C. Weitzman, "Access to Hospitals with High-Technology Cardiac Services: How is Race Important?" *American Journal of Public Health* 85, no. 3 (1995): 345–51.

6. Barnato and others, "Hospital-Level Racial Disparities," 308.

Chapter 6

1. Jonathan Klick and Thomas Stratmann, "Does Medical Malpractice Reform Help States Retain Physicians and Does it Matter?" Social Science Research Network, October 2, 2003, http://ssrn.com/abstract=453481 (accessed May 5, 2005).

2. Katherine Baicker and Amitabh Chandra, "The Productivity of Physician Specialization: Evidence from the Medicare Program," *American Economic Review* 94, no. 2 (2004): 357–61. The authors found that the doctors most sensitive to financial risks (those created by medical malpractice liability and, presumably, financial pressures in general) are those practicing in underserved areas.

3. Lisa Dubay, Robert Kaestner, and Timothy Waidmann, "Medical Malpractice Liability and Its Effect on Prenatal Care Utilization and Infant Health," *Journal of Health Economics* 20, no. 4 (2001): 591–611.

4. Daniel Kessler, William Sage, and David Becker, "Impact of Malpractice Reforms on the Supply of Physician Services," *The Journal of the American Medical Association* 293 (2005): 2618–25.

Chapter 7

1. Peter B. Bach and others, "Primary Care Physicians Who Treat Blacks and Whites," *New England Journal of Medicine* 351, no. 6 (2004): 575–84.

2. Eric C. Schneider, Alan M. Zaslavsky, and Arnold M. Epstein, "Racial Disparities in the Quality of Care for Enrollees in Medicare Managed Care," *The Journal of the American Medical Association* 287, no. 10 (2002): 1288–94.

3. Dana B. Mukamel, Ananthram S. Murthy, and David L. Weimer, "Racial Differences in Access to High-Quality Cardiac Surgeons," *American Journal of Public Health* 90, no. 11 (2000): 1774–77.

4. Barbara Rothenberg and others, "Explaining Disparities in Access to High-Quality Cardiac Surgeons," *Annals of Thoracic Surgery* 78 (2004): 18–25.

5. Donald Gemson, Jack Elinson, and Peter Messeri, "Differences in Physician Prevention Practice Patterns for White and Minority Patients," *Journal of Community Health* 13, no. 1 (1988): 53–64.

6. Kevin C. Heslin and others, "Racial and Ethnic Differences in Access to Physicians with HIV-Related Expertise," *Journal of General Internal Medicine* 20, no. 3 (2005): 283.

7. J. Lee Hargraves, Jeffrey J. Stoddard, and Sally Trude, "Minority Physicians' Experiences Obtaining Referrals to Specialists and Hospital Admissions," *Journal of General Medicine* 3, no. 3 (2001): 10.

Chapter 8

1. David R. Williams and Pamela Braboy Jackson, "Social Sources of Racial Disparities in Health," *Health Affairs* 24, no. 2 (2005): 325–34.

2. Isaacs and Schroeder, "Class—The Ignored Determinant"; John H. Stewart IV, "Carcinoma in African Americans: A Review of the Current Literature," *Cancer* 91, no. 12 (2001): 2476–82; Mitchell D. Wong and others, "Contribution of Major Diseases to Disparities in Mortality," *New England Journal of Medicine* 347, no. 20 (2002): 1585–92.

3. National Center for Health Statistics, "Prevalence of Overweight and Obesity among Adults in the United States," http://www.cdc.gov/nchs/products/pubs/pubd/hestats/3and4/overweight.htm (accessed July 26, 2005).

4. Mark S. Eberhardt and others, "Is Race Related to Glycemic Control? An Assessment of Glycosylated Hemoglobin in Two South Carolina Communities," *Journal of Clinical Epidemiology* 47, no. 10 (1994): 1181–89; Wendy F. Auslander and others, "Disparity in Glycemic Control and Adherence between African-American and Caucasian Youths with Diabetes: Family and Community Contexts," *Diabetes Care* 20, no. 10 (1997): 1569–75; Lorraine J. Weatherspoon and others, "Glycemic Control in a Sample of Black and White Clinic Patients with NIDDM," *Diabetes Care* 17, no. 10 (1994): 1148–53; Maureen I. Harris and others, "Racial and Ethnic Differences in Glycemic Control of Adults with Type 2 Diabetes," *Diabetes Care* 22, no. 3 (1999): 403–8; Ashwini Sehgal, "Impact of Quality Improvement Efforts on Race and Sex Disparities in Hemodialysis," *The Journal of the American Medical Association* 289, no. 8 (2003): 996–1000.

5. Williams and Jackson, "Social Sources of Racial Disparities."

6. Jeffrey A. Ferguson and others, "Examination of Racial Differences in Management of Cardiovascular Disease," *Journal of the American College of Cardiology* 30, no. 7 (1997): 1707–13.

7. Irwin S. Kirsch and others, *Adult Literacy in America: A First Look at the Findings of the National Adult Literacy Survey*, 3rd ed. (Washington, D.C.: National Center for Education, U.S. Department of Education, 2002), vol. 210, http://nces.ed.gov/pubs93/93275.pdf (accessed July 27, 2005).

8. Kitty S. Chan and others, "How Do Ethnicity and Primary Language Spoken at Home Affect Management Practices and Outcomes in Children and Adolescents with Asthma?" *Archives of Pediatric and Adolescent Medicine* 159, no. 3 (2005): 283–89.

9. Linda S Gottfredson "Intelligence: Is it the Epidemiologists' Elusive 'Fundamental Cause' of Social Class Inequalities in Health?" *Journal of Personality and Social Psychology* 86, no. 1 (2004): 174–199, available at http://www.udel.edu/educ/gottfredson/reprints/2004fundamentalcause.pdf (accessed November 22, 2005).

10. U.S. Department of Health and Human Services, Agency for Healthcare Research and Quality, "Literacy and Health Outcomes," *Evidence Report/Technology Assessment* no. 87, http://www.ahrq.gov/clinic/epcsums/litsum.htm (accessed August 29, 2005).

11. Institute of Medicine, *Health Literacy: A Prescription to End Confusion* (Washington, D.C.: National Academies Press, 2002), http://www.nap.edu/books/0309091179/html (accessed August 10, 2005).

12. Salam A. Ibrahim and others, "Understanding Ethnic Differences in the Utilization of Joint Replacement for Osteoarthritis: The Role of Patient-Level Factors," *Medical Care* 40, supp. 1 (2002): 144–51.

13. Mitchell L. Margolis and others, "Racial Differences Pertaining to a Belief About Lung Cancer Surgery: Results of a Multi-Center Study," *Annals of Internal Medicine* 139, no. 7 (2003): 558–63.

14. Jennifer McCann and others, "Evaluation of the Causes for Racial Disparity in Surgical Treatment of Early Stage Lung Cancer," *Chest* 128, no. 5 (2005): 3440–46.

15. Steven P. Sedlis and others, "Racial Differences in Performance of Invasive Cardiac Procedures in a Department of Veterans Affairs Medical Center," *Journal of Clinical Epidemiology* 50, no. 8 (1997): 899–901; Barnhart and others, "Clinical and Non-Clinical Correlates of Racial and Ethnic Differences."

16. Dana P. Goldman and James P. Smith, "Can Patient Self Management Help Explain the SES Health Gradient?" *Proceedings of the National Academy of Sciences* 99, no. 16 (1999): 10929–10934.

17. Ibid.

18. Russell L. Rothman and others, "Influence of Patient Literacy on the Effectiveness of a Primary Care-Based Diabetes Disease Management

Program," *The Journal of the American Medical Association* 292, no. 14 (2004): 1711–16.

Chapter 9

1. Sarah E. Brotherton, Paul H. Rockey, and Sylvia I. Etzel, "US Graduate Medical Education," *The Journal of the American Medical Association* 292, no. 9 (2004): 1032–37.

2. Brenda L. Beagan, "Teaching Social and Cultural Awareness to Medical Students: 'It's All Very Nice to Talk About it in Theory, But Ultimately it Makes No Difference,'" *Academic Medicine* 78, no. 6 (2003): 605.

3. Office of Minority Health, Assuring Cultural Competence in Health Care, "Recommendations for National Standards and an Outcomes-Focused Research Agenda," Standard 1, http://www.omhrc.gov/clas/finalcultural1a.htm#final1 (accessed June 4, 2005).

4. Liaison Committee on Medical Education, "Accreditation Standards to Obtaining an M.D. Degree," July 2003, www.lcme.org/functions2003july.pdf (accessed July 3, 2005).

5. Joseph R. Betancourt, "Cultural Competence—Marginal or Mainstream Movement?" *New England Journal of Medicine* 351, no. 10 (2004): 953.

6. Arthur Kleinman, "Culture and Depression," *New England Journal of Medicine* 351, no 10 (2004): 951–53. Kleinman reminds us that we cannot regard all Spanish-speakers as members of a homogenous group; there is considerable cultural variation among people from Cuba, Spain, Mexico, Nicaragua, and Puerto Rico, even though all speak a common language.

7. Alok A. Khorana, "Concordance," *Health Affairs* 24, no. 2 (2005): 511–15.

8. Bach and others, "Primary Care Physicians Who Treat Blacks and Whites."

9. Khorana, "Concordance."

10. Ibid., 514.

11. Ibid., 515.

12. Somnath Saha and others, "Do Patients Choose Physicians of Their Own Race? *Health Affairs* 19, no. 4 (2005): 76–83; Cohen, "The Consequences of Premature Abandonment of Affirmative Action."

13. Louis Harris and Associates, *Health Care Services and Minority Groups: A Comparative Survey of Whites, African-Americans, Hispanics and Asian-Americans*, study 932028 (New York: Commonwealth Fund, 1994), table 1-7.

14. Ibid., table 1-17.

15. Ibid., table 1-18.

16. Ibid., table 1-7.

17. Martha Harrison and Norman Thurston, "Racial Matching Among African Americans and Hispanic Physicians and Patients: Causes and Consequences," *Journal of Human Resources* 37, no. 2: 410–28; M. Komaromy and others, "The Role of Black and Hispanic Physicians in Providing Health Care for Underserved Populations," *New England Journal of Medicine* 334, no. 20 (May 16, 1996): 1305–10; H. K. Rabinowitz and others, "The Impact of Multiple Predictors on Generalist Physicians' Care of Underserved Populations," *American Journal of Public Health* 90, no. 8 (August 2000): 1225–28.

18. Ibid., table 4-10.

19. Ibid., table 3-27.

20. Ibid., table 4-10.

21. Ibid., table 4-14.

22. Ibid., table 4-10.

23. Ibid., table 1-3.

24. Frederick Schneiders Research, "Perceptions of How Race and Ethnic Background Affect Medical Care," focus group conducted for the Henry J. Kaiser Family Foundation, October 1999, 4.

25. Henry J. Kaiser Family Foundation, *Race, Ethnicity and Medical Care: A Survey of Public Perceptions and Experiences*, October 1999, 15. Also, even though 82 percent of African-Americans said their health care was excellent or good, 64 percent said they thought whites got better care than they did (9). See http://kaiseredu.org/topics_reflib.asp?id=329&parentid=67&rID=1(accessed October 7, 2005).

26. Ibid., 17.

27. Ibid., 22.

28. New America Wellness/Morehouse College of Medicine, Multiethnic Healthcare Attitudinal Research, research conducted by Erlich Transcultural Consultants, March 1999, available from Stedman Graham and Partners, New York. This finding correlated closely with the 27 percent of black respondents who did, in fact, have a black doctor. Only one in ten whites in this nationally representative sample expressed a preference for a white doctor, though the vast majority had one; Saha and others, "Do Patients Choose Physicians of Their Own Race?"; Cohen, "The Consequences of Premature Abandonment of Affirmative Action." In their paper, Saha and colleagues use 1994 Commonwealth data and report that a quarter of all black patients who saw a black doctor explicitly sought out a black physician. From this, the authors conclude that "minority patients choose physicians of their own race," 80. This conclusion does not seem warranted. Only one in four who already had a black doctor wanted one— not, seemingly, an overwhelming preference. Furthermore, 85 percent of black patients in the survey with white doctors had chosen them.

29. William D. King and others, "Does Racial Concordance Between HIV Positive Patients and Their Physicians Affect the Time to Receipt of Protease Inhibitors?" *Journal of General Internal Medicine* 19, no. 11 (2004): 1146–53 (found that black patients with white doctors were medicated over three months later than all other pairs); Thomas LaVeist, Amani Nuru-Jeter, and Kiesha Jones, "The Association of Doctor-Patient Race Concordance with Health Services Utilization," *Journal of Public Health Policy* 24, nos. 3–4 (2003): 312–23 (concordance mattered for whites and blacks but not for Hispanics and Asians); Somnath Saha, Jose J. Arbelaez, and Lisa A. Cooper, "Patient-Physician Relationship and Racial Disparities in the Quality of Health Care," *American Journal of Public Health* 93, no. 10 (2003): 1713–9 (found that concordance did not matter for services but had some effect on satisfaction); Trina Clark, Betsy Steath, and Richard H. Rubin, "Influence of Ethnicity and Language Concordance on Physician-Patient Agreement About Recommended Changes in Patient Health Behavior," *Patient Education and Counseling* 53, no. 1 (2004): 87–93 (found that concordance had no effect); Larry S. Wissow and others, "Longitudinal Care Lessens Differences in Mothers' Psychosocial Talk to Pediatricians Attributable to Ethnic and Gender Discordance," *Archives of Pediatrics and Adolescent Medicine* 157, no. 5 (2003): 419–24 (found that race-discordant pairs improved over course of year).

30. Mary Jo O'Sullivan and others, "Ethnic Populations: Community Mental Health Services Ten Years Later," *American Journal of Community Psychology* 17, no. 1 (1989): 17–30; Robert Rosenheck and Catherine L. Seibyl, "Participation and Outcome in a Residential Treatment and Work Therapy Program for Addictive Disorders: The Effects of Race," *The American Journal of Psychiatry* 155, no. 8 (1998): 1029–34; Stanley Sue and others, "Community Mental Health Services for Ethnic Minorities Groups: A Test of the Cultural Responsiveness Hypothesis," *American Psychologist* 59, no. 4 (1991): 533–40; Robert A. Rosenheck and Alan Fontana, "Race and Outcome of Treatment for Veterans Suffering from PTSD," *Journal of Traumatic Stress* 9, no. 2 (1996): 343–51; Robert A. Rosenheck and Alan Fontana, "Black and Hispanic Veterans in an Intensive VA Treatment Program for PTSD," *Medical Care* 40, suppl. I (2002): I52–61; Alexander N. Ortega and Robert A. Rosenheck, "Hispanic Client-Case Manager Matching: Differences in Outcomes and Service Use in a Program for Homeless Persons with Severe Mental Illness," *The Journal of Nervous and Mental Disease* 190, no. 5 (2002): 315–23 (patients in Hispanic pairing actually showed less improvement in psychosis than discordant pair); Catherine Leda and Robert A. Rosenheck, "Race in the Treatment of Homeless Mentally Ill Veterans," *The Journal of Nervous and Mental Disease* 183, no. 8 (1995): 529–33; Robert A. Rosenheck, Alan Fontana, and

Cheryl Cottrol, "Effect of Clinician-Veteran Racial Pairing in the Treatment of PTSD," *The American Journal of Psychiatry* 152, no. 4 (1995): 555–63. (On most measures, black patients performed equally irrespective of race of clinician; on a few, black patients did worse with white doctors than with black doctors.)

31. Matthew J. Chinman, Julie A. Lam, and Robert A. Rosenheck, "Clinician-Case Manager Racial Matching in a Program for Homeless Persons with Serious Mental Illness," *Psychiatric Services* 51, no. 10 (2000): 1265–72.

32. Thomas R. Konrad and others, "Physician-Patient Racial Concordance, Continuity of Care, and Patterns of Care for Hypertension," *American Journal of Public Health* 95, no.12 (2005): 2186–89.

33. Lisa Cooper-Patrick and others, "Race, Gender and Partnership in the Patient-Physician Relationship," *The Journal of the American Medical Association* 282, no. 6 (1999): 583–89. No data were provided to show whether patients' perceptions of being satisfied actually translated into objective measures of improved health, though it is well-established that a good rapport with one's doctor is associated with better treatment compliance.

34. These differences were statistically different; in a 2003 study, Cooper and colleagues found that concordance was associated with a longer visit, by two minutes, and an 8.4-point advantage in physician "participation." Yet an 8.0-point advantage is a rather small differential considering that the rating scale goes up to 120 possible points (mean for concordant pairs was 85 and for discordant 77). What's more, communication was rated as "patient-centered" irrespective of concordance; and, finally, no data on health outcomes were collected. Lisa A. Cooper and others, "Patient-Centered Communication, Ratings of Care, and Concordance of Patient and Physician Race," *Annals of Internal Medicine* 139, no. 11 (2003): 907–15.

35. Sherrie H. Kaplan and others, "Patient and Visit Characteristics Related to Physicians' Participatory Decision-Making Styles," *Medical Care* 33, no. 12 (1995): 1176–87.

36. Ibid.

37. Sherrie H. Kaplan and others, "Characteristics of Physicians with Participatory Decision-Making Styles," *Annals of Internal Medicine* 124, no. 5 (1996): 497–504.

38. Robert M. Kaplan, "Shared Decision Making: A New Tool for Preventative Medicine," *American Journal of Preventive Medicine* 26, no. 1 (2004): 67–80.

39. Lynn C. Smitherman, James Janisse, and Ambika Mathur, "Use of Folk Remedies Among Children in an Urban Black Community: Remedies for Fever, Colic and Teething," *Pediatrics* 115, no. 3 (2005): 297–304.

40. Donald R. Lannin and others, "Influence of Socioeconomic and Cultural Factors on Racial Differences in Late-Stage Presentation of Breast Cancer," *The Journal of the American Medical Association* 279, no. 22 (1998): 1801–07.

41. Sherrie Kaplan and Sheldon Greenfield, "The Patient's Role in Reducing Disparities," *Annals of Internal Medicine* 141, no. 3 (2004): 222–23.

42. Kathryn M. Rost and others, "Change in Metabolic Control and Functional Status after Hospitalization Impact of Patient Activation Intervention in Diabetic Patients," *Diabetes Care* 14, no. 10 (1991): 881–89; Lesley G. Frederikson and Peter E. Bull, "Evaluation of a Patient Education Leaflet Designed to Improve Communication in Medical Consultations," *Patient Education and Counseling* 25, no. 1 (February 1995): 51–57; Donald J. Cegala and others, "The Effects of Communication Skills Training on Patients' Participation during Medical Interviews," *Patient Education and Counseling* 41, no. 2 (2000): 209–22; Anh N. Tran and others, "Empowering Communication: A Community-Based Intervention for Patients," *Patient Education and Counseling* 52, no. 1 (January 2004): 113–21.

Conclusion

1. U.S. Department of Health and Human Services, Agency for Healthcare Research and Quality, "National Healthcare Disparities Report 2003," chap. 3, http://www.qualitytools.ahrq.gov/disparitiesreport/archive/2003/documents/3.quality_ss_0708.doc (accessed October 3, 2005).

2. Ibid., summary, http://www.ahrq.gov/qual/nhdr03/nhdrsum03.htm (accessed October 3, 2005).

3. Gilbert H. Friedell, MD (Director Emeritus, Markey Cancer Center, Lexington, Ky.), in discussion with authors, September 28, 2005.

4. William H. Frist, "Overcoming Disparities in U.S. Health Care," *Health Affairs* 24, no. 2 (2005): 445–51; Mark H. Showalter and Norman K. Thurston, "Taxes and Labor Supply of High-Income Physicians," *Journal of Public Economics* 66, no. 1 (1997): 73–97. The authors state that tax breaks are also an effective way to induce doctors to work more hours. This effect is especially strong with respect to solo practitioners. While these studies do not directly examine the willingness of doctors to practice in relatively unattractive areas, it seems likely that the income sensitivity they document would also apply to targeted payments to doctors that are made conditional on practicing in underserved areas.

5. For a definition of "usual source of care"—a commonly used measure of a person's ability to obtain high-quality care—see Nicole Lurie, "Measuring Disparities in Access to Care," in *IOM Guidelines for the National Healthcare Disparities Report*, ed. Elaine K. Swift (Washington, D.C.,

National Academies Press, 2000). Minorities are less likely to have a usual source of care (typically, meaning the same provider at each visit) than whites; this is strongly correlated with having health insurance, although insurance is not the only factor explaining racial differences in having a usual source of care. People with a regular source of care are more likely to obtain preventive and primary care; it may even be more important than insurance status in the receipt of health services; see Marsha Lillie-Blanton and Catherine Hoffman, "The Role of Health Insurance Coverage in Reducing Racial/Ethnic Disparities in Health Care," *Health Affairs* 24, no. 2 (2005): 398–408. See also Glorian Sorensen and others, "Promoting Behavior Change Among Working-Class, Multiethnic Workers: Results of the Health Directions-Small Business Study," *American Journal of Public Health* 95, no. 8 (2005): 1389–95; and Ann S. O'Malley and others, "Health Center Trends 1994–2001: What Do They Portend for the Federal Growth Initiative?" *Health Affairs* 24, no. 2 (2005): 465–72. O'Malley found that preventive service use shows negligible disparity between whites, blacks, and Hispanics. Harold P. Freeman, B. J. Muth, and Jon F. Kerner, "Expanding Access to Cancer Screening and Clinical Follow-Up among the Medically Underserved," *Cancer Practice* 3, no. 1 (1995): 19–30.

6. Of interest, "there is no empirical evidence that the power exerted on the doctor's communication behavior by [patient] narrative, questioning, expressions of concerns, and assertiveness differs by the patient's race or ethnicity," according to Carol Ashton and others, "Racial and Ethnic Disparities in the Use of Health Services: Bias, Preferences, or Poor Communication?" *Journal of General Internal Medicine* 18, no. 2 (2003): 146–52.

7. Isaacs and Schroeder, "Class—The Ignored Determinant."

8. Kathryn Baicker and Amitabh Chandra, "Medicare Spending, the Physician Workforce, and Beneficiaries' Quality of Care, *Health Affairs* supplemental web exclusive (2004): W184-97.

9. Amal N. Trivedi and others, *Trends in Quality of Care and Racial Disparities for Enrollees in Medicare Managed Care.*

10. J. Michael McGinnis, Pamela Williams-Russo, and James R. Knickman, "The Case for More Active Policy Attention to Health Promotion," *Health Affairs* 21, no. 2 (2002): 78–93, cited in Isaacs and Schroeder, "Class—The Ignored Determinant."

11. Avis J. Thomas and others, "Race/Ethnicity, Income, Major Risk Factors, and Cardiovascular Disease Mortality," *American Journal of Public Health* 95, no. 8 (2005): 1417–23.

About the Authors

Jonathan Klick is the Jeffrey A. Stoops Professor of Law at the Florida State University in Tallahassee, Florida, and an adjunct scholar at the American Enterprise Institute in Washington, D.C. Klick received his law degree and his PhD in economics from George Mason University. He has published widely about health care economics and issues related to individuals' access to care. He can be contacted at jklick@law.fsu.edu.

Sally L. Satel, MD, is a resident scholar at the American Enterprise Institute and the staff psychiatrist at the Oasis Clinic in Washington, D.C. She received a medical degree from Brown University and after completing her residency at Yale University School of Medicine, was an assistant professor of psychiatry at Yale from 1988 to 1993. From 1993 to 1994 she was a policy fellow with the Senate Labor and Human Resources Committee. She has written widely in academic journals on topics in psychiatry and medicine and has published articles on cultural aspects of medicine and science in numerous magazines and journals. Satel is author of *PC, M.D.: How Political Correctness Is Corrupting Medicine* (Basic Books, 2001), coauthor, with Nick Eberstadt, of *Health and Income Inequality: A Doctrine in Search of Data* (AEI Press, 2004), and coauthor, with Christina Hoff Sommers, of *One Nation Under Therapy* (St. Martin's Press, 2005).